IMAT Practice Papers

Volume Two

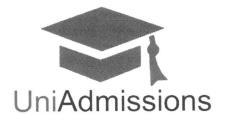

UniAdmissions

ISBN 978-1-912557-80-6

Published by *RAR Medical Services Limited*
www.uniadmissions.co.it
info@uniadmissions.co.it
Tel: 0208 068 0438

IMAT Practice Papers

4 Full Papers & Solutions

Alex Ochakovski
Rohan Agarwal

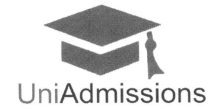

UniAdmissions

About the Authors

Alex is the co-founder and **Managing Director** at IMAT School, as well as the founder of MEDschool.it website. As a graduate of a first of a kind International Medical School in Italy, a former official supervisor of the IMAT test in Pavia and a dedicated curator of MEDschool.it, Alex has developed a deep understanding of the IMAT and the admission process over the years, following IMAT from the day it was created.

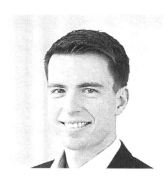

As an avid researcher with over ten peer-reviewed publications, experienced software developer, a fluent speaker of five languages and a medical doctor, Alex feels most fulfilled by combining his passions and strengths in projects that make a positive impact on society.

Thousands of current international medical students have been admitted to medical studies all over Italy with the help of the guidance and resources he provides to this day, creating a country-wide network of contacts in every International Medical School in Italy.

Rohan is the **Director of Operations** at *UniAdmissions* and is responsible for its technical and commercial arms. He graduated from Gonville and Caius College, Cambridge and is a fully qualified doctor. Over the last five years, he has tutored hundreds of successful Oxbridge and Medical applicants. He has also authored twenty books on admissions tests and interviews.

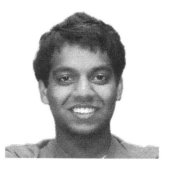

Rohan has taught physiology to undergraduate medical students and interviewed medical school applicants for Cambridge. He has published research on bone physiology and writes education articles for the Independent and Huffington Post. In his spare time, Rohan enjoys playing the piano and table tennis.

INTRODUCTION

The Basics

The International Medical Admissions Test (IMAT) is a 100-minute written exam for students who are applying to read medical and veterinary courses at competitive universities across the world.

It is a highly time pressured exam that forces you to apply knowledge in ways you have never thought about before. In this respect simply remembering solutions taught in class or from past papers is not enough.

However, fear not, despite what people say, you can actually prepare for the IMAT! With a little practice you can train your brain to manipulate and apply learnt methodologies to novel problems with ease. The best way to do this is through exposure to as many past/specimen papers as you can.

Preparing for the IMAT

Before going any further, it's important that you understand the optimal way to prepare for the IMAT. Rather than jumping straight into doing mock papers, it's essential that you start by understanding the components and the theory behind the IMAT by using an IMAT textbook. Once you've finished the non-timed practice questions, you can progress to past IMAT papers. These are freely available online at **www.uniadmissions.co.uk/IMAT-past-papers** and serve as excellent practice. You're strongly advised to use these in combination with the *IMAT Past Paper Worked Solutions* Book so that you can improve your weaknesses. Finally, once you've exhausted past papers, move onto the mock papers in this book.

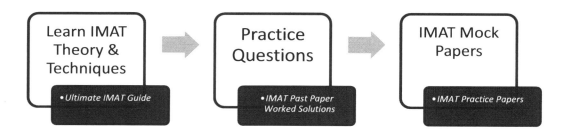

Already seen them all?

So, you've run out of past papers? Well hopefully that is where this book comes in. It contains eight unique mock papers; each compiled by expert IMAT tuors at *UniAdmissions* who scored in the top 10% nationally.

Having successfully gained a place on their course of choice, our tutors are intimately familiar with the IMAT and its associated admission procedures. So, the novel questions presented to you here are of the correct style and difficulty to continue your revision and stretch you to meet the demands of the IMAT.

General Advice

Start Early

It is much easier to prepare if you practice little and often. Start your preparation well in advance; ideally 10 weeks but at the latest within a month. This way you will have plenty of time to complete as many papers as you wish to feel comfortable and won't have to panic and cram just before the test, which is a much less effective and more stressful way to learn. In general, an early start will give you the opportunity to identify the complex issues and work at your own pace.

Prioritise

Some questions in sections can be long and complex – and given the intense time pressure you need to know your limits. It is essential that you don't get stuck with very difficult questions. If a question looks particularly long or complex, mark it for review and move on. You don't want to be caught 5 questions short at the end just because you took more than 3 minutes in answering a challenging multi-step question. If a question is taking too long, choose a sensible answer and move on. Remember that each question carries equal weighting and therefore, you should adjust your timing in accordingly. With practice and discipline, you can get very good at this and learn to maximise your efficiency.

Negative Marking

There is a penalty of -0.4 points for each incorrect answer in the IMAT. This removes the luxury of always being able to guess should you absolutely be not able to figure out the right answer for a question or run behind time. However this does not mean that you should not guess at all. Since each question provides you with 5 possible answers, you have a 20% chance of guessing correctly. Therefore, if you aren't sure (and are running short of time), try to eliminate a couple of answers to increase your chances of getting the question correct. For example, if a question has 5 options and you manage to eliminate 2 options- your chances of getting the question increase from 20% to 33%!

Practice

This is the best way of familiarising yourself with the style of questions and the timing for this section. Although the exam will essentially only test GCSE level knowledge, you are unlikely to be familiar with the style of questions in all sections when you first encounter them. Therefore, you want to be comfortable at using this before you sit the test.

Practising questions will put you at ease and make you more comfortable with the exam. The more comfortable you are, the less you will panic on the test day and the more likely you are to score highly. Initially, work through the questions at your own pace, and spend time carefully reading the questions and looking at any additional data. When it becomes closer to the test, **make sure you practice the questions under exam conditions**.

Past Papers

Official past papers and answers from 2011 onwards are freely available online on our website at www.uniadmissions.co.uk/IMAT-past-papers.

You will undoubtedly get stuck when doing some past paper questions – they are designed to be tricky and the answer schemes don't offer any explanations. Thus, **you're highly advised to acquire a copy of *IMAT Past Paper Worked Solutions*** – a free ebook is available online (see the back of this book for more details).

Repeat Questions

When checking through answers, pay particular attention to questions you have got wrong. If there is a worked answer, look through that carefully until you feel confident that you understand the reasoning, and then repeat the question without help to check that you can do it. If only the answer is given, have another look at the question and try to work out why that answer is correct. This is the best way to learn from your mistakes, and means you are less likely to make similar mistakes when it comes to the test. The same applies for questions which you were unsure of and made an educated guess which was correct, even if you got it right. When working through this book, **make sure you highlight any questions you are unsure of**, this means you know to spend more time looking over them once marked.

No Calculators

You aren't permitted to use calculators in the exam – thus, it is essential that you have strong numerical skills. For instance, you should be able to rapidly convert between percentages, decimals and fractions. You will seldom get questions that would require calculators, but you would be expected to be able to arrive at a sensible estimate. Consider for example:

Estimate 3.962 x 2.322;

3.962 is approximately 4 and 2.323 is approximately 2.33 = 7/3.

Thus, $3.962 \times 2.322 \approx 4 \times \frac{7}{3} = \frac{28}{3} = 9.33$

Since you will rarely be asked to perform difficult calculations, you can use this as a signpost of if you are tackling a question correctly. For example, when solving a physics question, you end up having to divide 8,079 by 357- this should raise alarm bells as calculations in the IMAT are rarely this difficult.

A word on timing...

"If you had all day to do your exam, you would get 100%. But you don't."
Whilst this isn't completely true, it illustrates a very important point. Once you've practiced and know how to answer the questions, the clock is your biggest enemy. This seemingly obvious statement has one very important consequence. **The way to improve your score is to improve your speed.** There is no magic bullet. But there are a great number of techniques that, with practice, will give you significant time gains, allowing you to answer more questions and score more marks.

Timing is tight throughout – **mastering timing is the first key to success**. Some candidates choose to work as quickly as possible to save up time at the end to check back, but this is generally not the best way to do it. Often questions can have a lot of information in them – each time you start answering a question it takes time to get familiar with the instructions and information. By splitting the question into two sessions (the first run-through and the return-to-check) you double the amount of time you spend on familiarising yourself with the data, as you have to do it twice instead of only once. This costs valuable time. In addition, candidates who do check back may spend 2–3 minutes doing so and yet not make any actual changes. Whilst this can be reassuring, it is a false reassurance as it is unlikely to have a significant effect on your actual score. Therefore, it is usually best to pace yourself very steadily, aiming to spend the same amount of time on each question and finish the final question in a section just as time runs out. This reduces the time spent on re-familiarising with questions and maximises the time spent on the first attempt, gaining more marks.

It is essential that you don't get stuck with the hardest questions – no doubt there will be some. In the time spent answering only one of these you may miss out on answering three easier questions. If a question is taking too long, choose a sensible answer and move on. Never see this as giving up or in any way failing, rather it is the smart way to approach a test with a tight time limit. With practice and discipline, you can get very good at this and learn to maximise your efficiency. It is not about being a hero and aiming for full marks – this is almost impossible and very much unnecessary (even Oxbridge will regard any score higher than 7 as exceptional). It is about maximising your efficiency and gaining the maximum possible number of marks within the time you have.

Use the Options:

Some questions may try to overload you with information. When presented with large tables and data, it's essential you look at the answer options so you can focus your mind. This can allow you to reach the correct answer a lot more quickly. Consider the example below:

The table below shows the results of a study investigating antibiotic resistance in staphylococcus populations. A single staphylococcus bacterium is chosen at random from a similar population. Resistance to any one antibiotic is independent of resistance to others.

Calculate the probability that the bacterium selected will be resistant to all four drugs.

A   1 in 10^6
B   1 in 10^{12}
C   1 in 10^{20}
D   1 in 10^{25}
E   1 in 10^{30}
F   1 in 10^{35}

Antibiotic	Number of Bacteria tested	Number of Resistant Bacteria
Benzyl-penicillin	10^{11}	98
Chloramphenicol	10^9	1200
Metronidazole	10^8	256
Erythromycin	10^5	2

Looking at the options first makes it obvious that there is **no need to calculate exact values**- only in powers of 10. This makes your life a lot easier. If you hadn't noticed this, you might have spent well over 90 seconds trying to calculate the exact value when it wasn't even being asked for.

In other cases, you may actually be able to use the options to arrive at the solution quicker than if you had tried to solve the question as you normally would. Consider the example below:

A region is defined by the two inequalities: $x - y^2 > 1 \; and \; xy > 1$. Which of the following points is in the defined region?

A.   (10,3)
B.   (10,2)
C.   (-10,3)
D.   (-10,2)
E.   (-10,-3)

Whilst it's possible to solve this question both algebraically or graphically by manipulating the identities, by far **the quickest way is to actually use the options**. Note that options C, D and E violate the second inequality, narrowing down to answer to either A or B. For A: $10 - 3^2 = 1$ and thus this point is on the boundary of the defined region and not actually in the region. Thus the answer is B (as $10-4 = 6 > 1$.)

In general, it pays dividends to look at the options briefly and see if they can be help you arrive at the question more quickly. Get into this habit early – it may feel unnatural at first but it's guaranteed to save you time in the long run.

Keywords

If you're stuck on a question; pay particular attention to the options that contain key modifiers like "**always**", "**only**", "**all**" as examiners like using them to test if there are any gaps in your knowledge. E.g. the statement "arteries carry oxygenated blood" would normally be true; "All arteries carry oxygenated blood" would be false because the pulmonary artery carries deoxygenated blood.

Manage your Time:

It is highly likely that you will be juggling your revision alongside your normal school studies. Whilst it is tempting to put your A-levels on the back burner falling behind in your school subjects is not a good idea, don't forget that to meet the conditions of your offer should you get one you will need at least one A*. So, time management is key!

Make sure you set aside a dedicated 90 minutes (and much more once you're closer to the exam) to commit to your revision each day. The key here is not to sacrifice too many of your extracurricular activities, everybody needs some down time, but instead to be efficient. Take a look at our list of top tips for increasing revision efficiency below:

1. Create a comfortable work station
2. Declutter and stay tidy
3. Treat yourself to some nice stationery
4. See if music works for you → if not, find somewhere peaceful and quiet to work
5. Turn off your mobile or at least put it into silent mode
6. Silence social media alerts
7. Keep the TV off and out of sight
8. Stay organised with to do lists and revision timetables – more importantly, stick to them!
9. Keep to your set study times and don't bite off more than you can chew
10. Study while you're commuting
11. Adopt a positive mental attitude
12. Get into a routine
13. Consider forming a study group to focus on the harder exam concepts
14. Plan rest and reward days into your timetable – these are excellent incentive for you to stay on track with your study plans!

Keep Fit & Eat Well:

'A car won't work if you fill it with the wrong fuel' - your body is exactly the same. You cannot hope to perform unless you remain fit and well. The best way to do this is not underestimate the importance of healthy eating. Beige, starchy foods will make you sluggish; instead start the day with a hearty breakfast like porridge. Aim for the recommended 'five a day' intake of fruit/veg and stock up on the oily fish or blueberries – the so called "super foods".

When hitting the books, it's essential to keep your brain hydrated. If you get dehydrated you'll find yourself lethargic and possibly developing a headache, neither of which will do any favours for your revision. Invest in a good water bottle that you know the total volume of and keep sipping through the day. Don't forget that the amount of water you should be aiming to drink varies depending on your mass, so calculate your own personal recommended intake as follows: 30 ml per kg per day.

It is well known that exercise boosts your wellbeing and instils a sense of discipline. All of which will reflect well in your revision. It's well worth devoting half an hour a day to some exercise, get your heart rate up, break a sweat, and get those endorphins flowing.

Sleep

It's no secret that when revising you need to keep well rested. Don't be tempted to stay up late revising as sleep actually plays an important part in consolidating long term memory. Instead aim for a minimum of 7 hours good sleep each night, in a dark room without any glow from electronic appliances. Install flux (https://justgetflux.com) on your laptop to prevent your computer from disrupting your circadian rhythm. Aim to go to bed the same time each night and no hitting snooze on the alarm clock in the morning!

Revision Timetable

Still struggling to get organised? Then try filling in the example revision timetable below, remember to factor in enough time for short breaks, and stick to it! Remember to schedule in several breaks throughout the day and actually use them to do something you enjoy e.g. TV, reading, YouTube etc.

	8AM	0AM		2PM	4PM	6PM	3PM
MONDAY							
TUESDAY							
HURSDAY							
FRIDAY							
ATURDAY							
SUNDAY							
EXAMPLE DAY	School			Biology	Problem	vsics	

ou have a much more accurate idea of the time you're spending on a question. In general, if you've spent >150 conds on a section 1 question or >90 seconds on a section 2 questions – move on regardless of how close you think you are to solving it.

Getting the most out of Mock Papers

Mock exams can prove invaluable if tackled correctly. Not only do they encourage you to start revision earlier, they also allow you to **practice and perfect your revision technique**. They are often the best way of improving your knowledge base or reinforcing what you have learnt. Probably the best reason for attempting mock papers is to familiarise yourself with the exam conditions of the IMAT as they are particularly tough.

Start Revision Earlier

Thirty five percent of students agree that they procrastinate to a degree that is detrimental to their exam performance. This is partly explained by the fact that they often seem a long way in the future. In the scientific literature this is well recognised, Dr. Piers Steel, an expert on the field of motivation states that *'the further away an event is, the less impact it has on your decisions'*.

Mock exams are therefore a way of giving you a target to work towards and motivate you in the run up to the real thing – every time you do one treat it as the real deal! If you do well then it's a reassuring sign; if you do poorly then it will motivate you to work harder (and earlier!).

Practice and perfect revision techniques

In case you haven't realised already, revision is a skill all to itself, and can take some time to learn. For example, the most common revision techniques including **highlighting and/or re-reading are quite ineffective** ways of committing things to memory. Unless you are thinking critically about something you are much less likely to remember it or indeed understand it.

Mock exams, therefore allow you to test your revision strategies as you go along. Try spacing out your revision sessions so you have time to forget what you have learnt in-between. This may sound counterintuitive but the second time you remember it for longer. Try teaching another student what you have learnt, this forces you to structure the information in a logical way that may aid memory. Always try to question what you have learnt and appraise its validity. Not only does this aid memory but it is also a useful skill for IMAT section 3, Oxbridge interview, and beyond.

Improve your knowledge

The act of applying what you have learnt reinforces that piece of knowledge. A question may ask you to think about a relatively basic concept in a novel way (not cited in textbooks), and so deepen your understanding. Exams rarely test word for word what is in the syllabus, so when running through mock papers try to understand how the basic facts are applied and tested in the exam. As you go through the mocks or past papers take note of your performance and see if you consistently under-perform in specific areas, thus highlighting areas for future study.

Get familiar with exam conditions

Pressure can cause all sorts of trouble for even the most brilliant students. The IMAT is a particularly time pressured exam with high stakes – your future (without exaggerating) does depend on your result to a great extent. The real key to the IMAT is overcoming this pressure and remaining calm to allow you to think efficiently.

Mock exams are therefore an excellent opportunity to devise and perfect your own exam techniques to beat the pressure and meet the demands of the exam. **Don't treat mock exams like practice questions – it's imperative you do them under time conditions.**

emember! It's better that you make all the mistakes you possibly can now in mock papers and then learn om them so as not to repeat them in the real exam.

Things to have done before using this book

Do the ground work
- Read in detail: the background, methods, and aims of the IMAT as well logistical considerations such as how to take the IMAT in practice. A good place to start is a IMAT textbook like *The Ultimate IMAT Guide* (flick to the back to get a free copy!) which covers all the groundwork but it's also worth looking through the official IMAT site (www.admissionstesting.org/IMAT).
- It is generally a good idea to start re-capping all your GCSE maths and science.
- Practice substituting formulas together to reach a more useful one expressing known variables e.g. $P = IV$ and $V = IR$ can be combined to give $P = V^2/R$ and $P = I^2R$. Remember that calculators are not permitted in the exam, so get comfortable doing more complex long addition, multiplication, division, and subtraction.
- Get comfortable rapidly converting between percentages, decimals, and fractions.
- Practice developing logical arguments and structuring essays with an obvious introduction, main body, and ending.
- These are all things which are easiest to do alongside your revision for exams before the summer break. Not only gaining a head start on your IMAT revision but also complimenting your year 12 studies well.
- Discuss scientific problems with others - propose experiments and state what you think the result would be. Be ready to defend your argument. This will rapidly build your scientific understanding for section 2 but also prepare you well for an oxbridge interview.
- Read through the IMAT syllabus before you start tackling whole papers. This is absolutely essential. It contains several stated formulae, constants, and facts that you are expected to apply - or may just be an answer in their own right. Familiarising yourself with the syllabus is also a quick way of teaching yourself the additional information other exam boards may learn which you do not. Sifting through the whole IMAT syllabus is a time-consuming process so we have done it for you. **Be sure to flick through the syllabus checklist** later on, which also doubles up as a great revision aid for the night before!

Ease in gently
With the ground work laid, there's still no point in adopting exam conditions straight away. Instead invest in a beginner's guide to the IMAT, which will not only describe in detail the background and theory of the exam, but take you through section by section what is expected. *The Ultimate IMAT Guide: 800 Practice Questions* is the most popular IMAT textbook – you can get a free copy by flicking to the back of this book.

When you are ready to move on to past papers, take your time and puzzle your way through all the questions. Really try to understand solutions. A past paper question won't be repeated in your real exam, so don't rote learn methods or facts. Instead, focus on applying prior knowledge to formulate your own approach.

If you're really struggling and have to take a sneak peek at the answers, then practice thinking of alternative solutions, or arguments for essays. It is unlikely that your answer will be more elegant or succinct than the model answer, but it is still a good task for encouraging creativity with your thinking. Get used to thinking outside the box!

Accelerate and Intensify

Start adopting exam conditions after you've done two past papers. Don't forget that **it's the time pressure that makes the IMAT hard** – if you had as long as you wanted to sit the exam you would probably get 100%. If you're struggling to find comprehensive answers to past papers then *IMAT Past Papers Worked Solutions* contains detailed explained answers to every IMAT past paper question and essay (flick to the back to get a free copy).

Doing all the past papers from 2009 – present is a good target for your revision. Note that the IMAT syllabus changed in 2009 so questions before this date may no longer be relevant. In any case, choose a paper and proceed with strict exam conditions. Take a short break and then mark your answers before reviewing your progress. For revision purposes, as you go along, keep track of those questions that you guess – these are equally as important to review as those you get wrong.

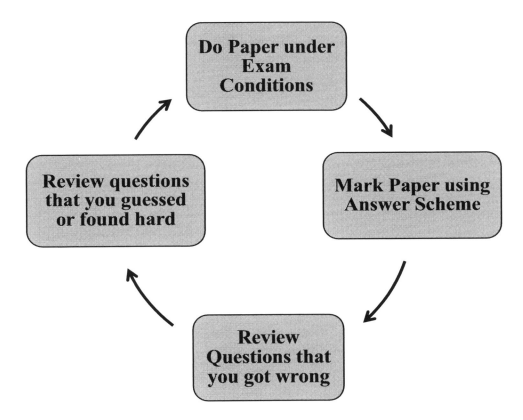

Once you've exhausted all the past papers, move on to tackling the unique mock papers in this book. In general, you should aim to complete one to two mock papers every night in the ten days preceding your exam.

Section 1: An Overview

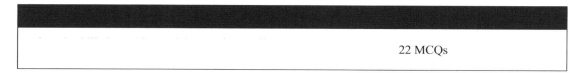

22 MCQs

This is the first section of the IMAT, comprising what most people describe as the classic IQ test style questions. Giving you one hour to answer 35 questions testing your ability to think critically, solve problems, and handle data. Breaking things down you realise that you are left with approximately 100 seconds per question. Remember though that this not only includes reasoning your answers, but also reading passages of text and/or analysing diagrams or graphs.

Not all the questions are of equal difficulty and so as you work through the past material it is certainly worth learning to recognise quickly which questions you need to skip to avoid getting bogged down. If it comes to it and you do not have enough time to go back to any skipped questions at the end, you always have a 20% chance of getting the answer correct with a guess!

Critical thinking questions
These types of question will generally present you with a passage of text or a methodology for an experiment and ask you to do one of three things: identify a conclusion, identify and assumption or flaw, or give an argument to either strengthen or weaken the statement.

The ability to filter through irrelevant material is essential with these questions as well as a solid grasp of the English language. Remember to only use the information given to you in your reasoning and never be too general with your conclusions – seek direct evidence in the information given. Critical thinking questions are definitely an example of when it is **best to read the question first**!

Problem solving questions
The problems in section 1 are often very wordy and complex, therefore it is often useful to turn the prose of the question into a series of equations. For example, being able to turn the sentence "Megan is half as tall as Elin" into "2M = E" should become second nature to you. Trial and error is not a method you should adopt for any questions in section 1 as it is far too time consuming.

As you are working through the preparation material try to get used to recognising which questions can be aided by drawing a quick diagram. This could apply to questions asking about timetables, orders, sequences, or spatial relationships. Remember it doesn't have to be pretty, merely help you organise your thoughts!

Data handling questions
These questions will undoubtedly require you to work with numbers, often calculating percentages or frequencies. Again, reading the question first can help you save time here, directing your attention to the relevant information in the passage. When analysing tables or graphs always check the following:

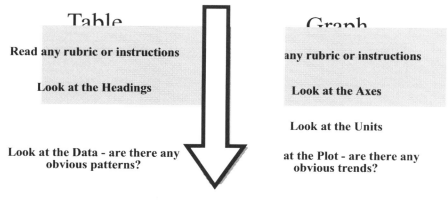

Sections 2, 3 & 4: An Overview

What will you be tested on?	No. of Questions	Duration
Ability to recall, understand and apply scientific knowledge and principles of biology, chemistry, physics, and maths. Usually the sections that students find the hardest.	38 MCQs	65 Minutes

If you're short of time, then these sections are where to focus. Undoubtedly the most time pressured section of the IMAT (requiring you to answer a question every 100 seconds) but also the section where candidates improve the fastest. These sections draw on your knowledge of biology, chemistry, physics, and maths.

Biology

Generally, the biology questions require the least amount of time and are often where you can rely on making up lost time from harder questions. Most of biology questions rely on you being able to recall facts rather than interpret data or solve equations, so some good old-fashioned text book revision will prepare you well for these questions.

Chemistry

If you're taking the IMAT you will undoubtedly be studying chemistry at A-level as it is a requirement of all medical schools. Conceptually therefore, you should be in the clear, however, balancing complex equations or processing lengthy calculations can be time consuming.

Practicing with mock papers is essentially in combating this – really focus on extracting what the question is asking for as quickly as possible. In addition to the equations on the subsequent pages you must be comfortable with converting between litres, dm^3, cm^3, and mm^3 as well as using Avogadro's constant in calculations.

Physics

Physics is by far the most common subject that students drop moving on to AS-level, meaning these questions are the most poorly answered. There is a large variation in physics specifications between GCSE exam boards, so **before you do anything else read through the IMAT syllabus and commit all the stated equations and constants to memory** (helpfully highlighted in bold type on the revision checklist).

Physics questions will almost always require a two-step solution, normally forcing you to combine and re-arrange equations. All answers must be given in SI units which actually benefits you, by looking at the units you can often derive the equation – for example speed in m/s is calculated as distance(m) / time(s). It is also worth becoming fluent with the terminology for orders of magnitude in measurements (see right).

Maths

Maths is the single most important component of section 2, a question topic in its own right but also applied in chemistry, physics, and section 1. Just remember to limit yourself to GCSE knowledge in the maths questions and don't overcomplicate things. As a bare minimum for preparation you should practice applying the quadratic formula, completing the square, and finding the difference between 2 squares.

Factor	Text	Symbol
10^{12}	Tera	T
10^{9}	Giga	G
10^{6}	Mega	M
10^{3}	Kilo	k
10^{2}	Hecto	h
10^{-1}	Deci	d
10^{-2}	Centi	c
10^{-3}	Milli	m
10^{-6}	Micro	μ
10^{-9}	Nano	n
10^{-12}	Pico	p

How to use this Book

If you have done everything this book has described so far then you should be well equipped to meet the demands of the IMAT, and therefore **the mock papers in the rest of this book should ONLY be completed under exam conditions**.

This means:

➢ Absolute silence – no TV or music
➢ Absolute focus – no distractions such as eating your dinner
➢ Strict time constraints – no pausing half way through
➢ No checking the answers as you go
➢ Give yourself a maximum of three minutes between sections – keep the pressure up
➢ Complete the entire paper before marking
➢ Mark harshly

In practice this means setting aside two hours in an evening to find a quiet spot without interruptions and tackle the paper. Completing one mock paper every evening in the week running up to the exam would be an ideal target.

➢ Tackle the paper as you would in the exam.
➢ Return to mark your answers, but mark harshly if there's any ambiguity.
➢ Highlight any areas of concern.
➢ If warranted read up on the areas you felt you underperformed to reinforce your knowledge.
➢ If you inadvertently learnt anything new by muddling through a question, go and tell somebody about it to reinforce what you've discovered.

Finally relax… the IMAT is an exhausting exam, concentrating so hard continually for two hours will take its toll. So, being able to relax and switch off is essential to keep yourself sharp for exam day! Make sure you reward yourself after you finish marking your exam.

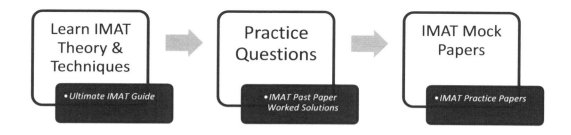

Scoring Tables

Use these to keep a record of your scores from past papers – you can then easily see which paper you should attempt next (always the one with the lowest score).

SECTION 1	1st Attempt	2nd Attempt	3rd Attempt
2011			
2012			
2013			
2014			
2015			
2016			
2017			
2018			

SECTION 2	1st Attempt	2nd Attempt	3rd Attempt
2011			
2012			
2013			
2014			
2015			
2016			
2017			
2018			

SECTION 3	1st Attempt	2nd Attempt	3rd Attempt
2011			
2012			
2013			
2014			
2015			
2016			
2017			
2018			

SECTION 4	1st Attempt	2nd Attempt	3rd Attempt
2011			
2012			
2013			
2014			
2015			
2016			
2017			
2018			

And the same again here but with our mocks instead.

SECTION 1	1st Attempt	2nd Attempt	3rd Attempt
Mock E			
Mock F			
Mock G			
Mock H			

SECTION 2	1st Attempt	2nd Attempt	3rd Attempt
Mock E			
Mock F			
Mock G			
Mock H			

SECTION 3	1st Attempt	2nd Attempt	3rd Attempt
Mock E			
Mock F			
Mock G			
Mock H			

SECTION 4	1st Attempt	2nd Attempt	3rd Attempt
Mock E			
Mock F			
Mock G			
Mock H			

MOCK PAPER E

Section 1

Question 1:
What is the capital of Brazil?

A) Rio De Janiero
B) Brasilia
C) Begota
D) Sao Paolo
E) Buenos Aires

Question 2:
Which two philosophers wrote the Communist manifesto together?

A) Marx and Hegel
B) Marx and schiller
C) Marx and Engels
D) Marx and Frege
E) Hegel and Schiller

Question 3:
The Minoan Civilisation was on what Mediterranean Island?

A) Crete
B) Malta
C) Cyprus
D) Sardinia
E) Rhodes

Question 4:
Occam's razor is the philosophical principle that given two explanations for something which is preferred?

A) The longest
B) The most complex
C) The simplest
D) The most optimistic
E) The most radical

Question 5:
Which English Romantic poet wrote the line 'I wandered lonely as a cloud'?

A) Keats
B) Wordsworth
C) Shakespeare
D) John Donne
E) Byron

Question 6:

Which American politician was controversially awarded the Nobel peace prize for his dealings in the Vietnam war?

A) Henry Kissinger
B) Richard Nixon
C) Dick Cheney
D) Gerald Ford
E) Alan Greenspan

Question 7:
Which British political party was founded in 1900?

A) Labour
B) Conservative
C) Whig
D) Green
E) Liberal

Question 8:
In Computing what is the name give to the central component inside the computer?

A) Mainframe
B) Hub
C) Megatron
D) Mediacentre
E) Motherboard

Question 9:
Lord Admiral Nelson died during which battle?

A) Lepranto
B) Waterloo
C) Trafalgar
D) Balfour
E) St Petersburg

Question 10:
Steve Jobs founded what company in 1976?

A) Apple
B) Microsoft
C) IBM
D) Tinder
E) Pixar

Question 11:
Which philosophers' *Meditations*, published in 1641 contained the famous maxim 'I think therefore I am'

A) Rene Descartes
B) Roger Bacon
C) Aristotle
D) Plato
E) Frederic Nietzsche

Question 12:

Which painter painted the Sistine chapel?

A) Leonardo Da Vinci
B) Michelangelo
C) Botticelli
D) Rembrandt
E) Gustav Klimt

Question 13:
Hannah, Jane and Tom are travelling to London to see a musical. Hannah catches the train at 1430. Jane leaves at the same time as Hannah, but catches a bus which takes 40% longer then Hannah's train. Tom also takes a train, and the journey time is 10 minutes less then Hannah's journey, but he leaves 45 minutes after Jane leaves. He arrives in London at 1620.

At what time will Jane arrive in London?

A) 1545   B) 1600   C) 1615   D) 1700   E) 1715

Question 14:
At a show, there are two different ticket prices for different seats. The cost is £10 for a standard seat, and £16 for a premium view seat. The total revenue from a show is £6,600, and the total attendance was 600.

How many premium view seats were purchased?

A) 60   B) 100   C) 140   D) 180   E) 240

Question 15:
The moon orbits the Earth once every 28 days. Between 20th January and 23rd May inclusive, how many degrees has the Moon turned through? This is not a leap year.

A) 1540°   B) 1560°   C) 1580°   D) 1600°   E) 1620°

Question 16:
Drama academies are special schools students can go to in order to learn performing arts. These schools are only available to the most skilled young performers, and aim to give students the best training in the arts, whilst still covering mainstream academic subjects. However, many parents are reluctant for their children to attend such academies, as they feel the academic teaching will be worse than at a standard school.

Which of the following, if true, would most weaken the above argument?

A) Most top actors attended a drama academy as children
B) There is as much time dedicated to academic work in drama academies as there is in normal schools
C) The academic work comprises a greater proportion of the study time than drama related activities
D) Most children are keen to attend a drama academy if given the opportunity
E) 80% of students at drama academies attain higher than average GCSE scores

Question 17:
Anil and Suresh both leave point A at the same time. Anil travels 5km East then 10km North. Anil then travels a further 1km North before heading 3km West. Suresh travels East for 2km less than Anil's total journey distance. He then heads 13km North, before pausing and travelling back 2km South. How far, as the crow flies, are the two men now apart?

A) 11km   B) 12km   C) 13km   D) 15km   E) 17km

Question 18:
Chris leaves his house to go and visit Laura, who lives 3 miles away. He leaves at 1730 and walks at 4mph towards Laura's house, stopping for one 5-minute to chat to a friend. Meanwhile Sarah also wants to visit Laura. She sets off from her house 6 miles away at 1810, driving in her car and averaging a speed of 24mph.

Who reaches the house first and with how long do they wait for the other person?

A) Chris, and waits 5 mins for Sarah   D) Sarah, and waits 10 mins for Chris
B) Chris, and waits 10 mins for Sarah   E) They both arrive at the same time
C) Sarah, and waits 5 mins for Chris

Question 19:
 "Illegal film and music downloads have increased greatly in recent years. This causes significant harm to the relevant industries. Many people justify this to themselves by telling themselves they are only diverting money away from wealthy and successful singers and actors, who do not need any more money anyway. But in reality, illegal downloads are deeply harming the music industry, making many studio workers redundant and making it difficult for less famous performers to make a living."

Which of the following best summarises the conclusion of this argument?

A) Unemployment is a problem in the music industry
B) Taking profits away from successful musicians does more harm than good
C) Studio workers are most affected by illegal downloads
D) Illegal downloads cause more harm than people often think
E) Buying music legally helps keep the music industry productive

Question 20:
"40,000 litres of water will extinguish two typical house fires. 70,000 litres of water will extinguish two house fires and three garden fires. There is no surplus water"

Which statement is **NOT** true?

A) A garden fire can be extinguished with 12,000 litres, with water to spare.
B) 20,000 litres is sufficient to extinguish a normal house fire.
C) A garden fire requires only half as much water to extinguish as a house fire.
D) Two house and four garden fires will need 80,000 litres to extinguish.
E) Three house and ten garden fires will need 140,000 litres to extinguish.

Question 21:
"Plans are in place to install antennas underground, so that users of underground trains will be able to pick up mobile reception. There are, as usual, winners and losers from this policy. Supporters of the policy argue that it will lead to an increase in workforce productivity and increase convenience in day-to-day life. Critics respond by saying that it will lead to an annoying environment whilst travelling, it will facilitate the ease of conducting a terrorist threat and it will decrease levels of sociability. The latter camp seems to have the greatest support and so a re-consideration of the policy is urged."

Which of the following **best** summarises the conclusion of this passage?

A) The disadvantages of installing underground antennas outweigh the benefits
B) The cost of the scheme is likely to be prohibitive
C) The policy must be dropped, since a majority does not want it
D) More people don't want this scheme than do want it
E) A detailed consultation process should take place

Question 22:
"Ecosystems in the oceans are changing. Recently, restrictions on fishing have been imposed to tackle the decline in fish populations. As a result, farm fishing and the price of fish have increased, whilst the seas recover. It is hoped that these changes will lead to a brighter future for all."

Which of the following are **TWO** assumptions of this argument?

A) People will still buy farmed fish at a higher price
B) The population of wild fish can recover
C) Fishermen will benefit from working on this scheme
D) Ecosystems have been altered as a result of climate change
E) Heavy sea fishing is to blame for the changes in the ecosystem

END OF SECTION

Section 2

Question 23:
Which of the following statements, regarding normal human digestion, is **FALSE**?

A) Amylase is an enzyme which breaks down starch
B) Amylase is produced by the pancreas
C) Bile is stored in the gallbladder
D) The small intestine is the longest part of the gut
E) Insulin is released in response to feeding
F) None of the above

Question 24:
Jane is one mile into a marathon. Which of the following statements is **NOT** true, relative to before she started?

A) Blood flow to the skin is increased
B) Blood flow to the muscles is increased
C) Blood flow to the gut is decreased
D) Blood flow to the kidneys is decreased
E) Cardiac Output Increases
F) None of the above

Question 25:
A newly discovered species of beetle is found to have 29.6% Adenine (A) bases in its genome. What is the percentage of Cytosine (C) bases in the beetle's DNA?

A) 20.4%
B) 29.6%
C) 40.8%
D) 59.2%
E) 70.6%
F) More information is required

Question 26:
Carbon monoxide binds irreversibly to the oxygen binding site of haemoglobin. Which of the following statements is true regarding carbon monoxide poisoning?

A) Carbon monoxide poisoning has no serious consequences
B) Haemoglobin is heavier, as both oxygen and carbon monoxide bind to it
C) Affected individuals have a raised heart rate
D) The CO_2 carrying capacity of the blood is decreased
E) The O_2 carrying capacity of the blood is unchanged as it dissolves in the plasma instead

Question 27:
Antibiotics can have serious side effects such as liver failure and renal failure. Therefore, scientists are always trying to develop antibiotics to minimise these effects by targeting specific cellular components. Which of these cellular components offers the best way to treat infections and minimise side effects?

A) Mitochondrion
B) Cell membrane
C) Nucleic acid
D) Cytoskeleton
E) Flagellum

Question 28:
Study the following diagram of the human heart. What is true about structure **A**?

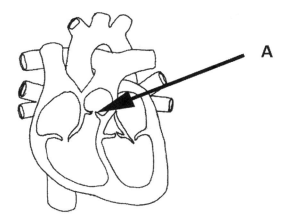

A) It is closed during systole
B) It prevents blood flowing into the left ventricle during systole
C) It prevents blood flowing into the right ventricle during systole
D) It prevents blood flowing into the left ventricle during diastole
E) It opens due to left ventricular pressure being greater than aortic pressure.
F) It is open when the right ventricle is emptying

Question 29:
A person responds to the starting gun of a race and begins to run. Place the following order of events in the most likely chronological sequence. Which option is a correct sequence?

1   Blood CO_2 increases

2   The eardrum vibrates to the sound

3   Impulses travel along motor neurones

4   Impulses travel along sensory neurones

5   Impulses travel along relay neurones

6   Quadriceps muscles contract

7   Glycogen is converted into glucose

8   Creatine phosphate rapidly re-phosphorylates ADP

A) $2 \rightarrow 5 \rightarrow 4 \rightarrow 3 \rightarrow 6 \rightarrow 7$
B) $2 \rightarrow 4 \rightarrow 3 \rightarrow 8 \rightarrow 6 \rightarrow 1$
C) $2 \rightarrow 3 \rightarrow 4 \rightarrow 6 \rightarrow 7 \rightarrow 1$
D) $2 \rightarrow 4 \rightarrow 3 \rightarrow 1 \rightarrow 6 \rightarrow 7$
E) $2 \rightarrow 4 \rightarrow 3 \rightarrow 6 \rightarrow 8 \rightarrow 7$

Question 30:
Which of the following best describes the events that occur during expiration?

A) The ribs move up and in; the diaphragm moves down.
B) The ribs move down and in; the diaphragm moves up.
C) The ribs move up and in; the diaphragm moves up.
D) The ribs move down and out; the diaphragm moves down.
E) The ribs move up and out; the diaphragm moves down.
F) The ribs move up and out; the diaphragm moves up.

Question 31:
Vijay goes to see his GP with fatty, smelly stools that float on water. Which of the following enzymes is most likely to be malfunctioning?

A) Amylase   B) Lipase   C) Protease   D) Sucrase   E) Lactase

Question 32:
Which of the following statements concerning the cardiovascular system is correct?

A) Oxygenated blood from the lungs flows to the heart via the pulmonary artery.
B) All arteries carry oxygenated blood.
C) All animals have a double circulatory system.
D) The superior vena cava contains oxygenated blood
E) All veins have valves.
F) None of the above.

Question 33:
Which part of the GI tract has the least amount of enzymatic digestion occurring?

A) Mouth   C) Small intestine   E) Rectum
B) Stomach   D) Large intestine

Question 34:
Oge touches a hot stove and immediately moves her hand away. Which of the following components are **NOT** involved in this reaction?

1. Thermo-receptor   3. Spinal Cord   5. Motor nerve
2. Brain   4. Sensory nerve   6. Muscle

A) 1 only   C) 3 only   E) 1, 2 and 3 only
B) 2 only   D) 1 and 2 only   F) 3, 4, 5 and 6

Question 35:
Which of the following represents a scenario with an appropriate description of the mode of transport?

1. Water moving from a hypotonic solution outside of a potato cell, across the cell wall and cell membrane and into the hypertonic cytoplasm of the potato cell→ Osmosis.
2. Carbon dioxide moving across a respiring cell's membrane and dissolving in blood plasma →Active transport.
3. Reabsorption of amino acids against a concentration gradient in the glomeruluar apparatus → Diffusion.

A) 1 only   C) 3 only   E) 2 and 3 only   G) 1, 2 and 3
B) 2 only   D) 1 and 2 only   F) 1 and 3 only

Question 36:
Which of the following equations represents anaerobic respiration?

1.   Carbohydrate + Oxygen → Energy + Carbon Dioxide + Water
2.   Carbohydrate → Energy + Lactic Acid + Carbon dioxide
3.   Carbohydrate → Energy + Lactic Acid
4.   Carbohydrate → Energy + Ethanol + Carbon dioxide

A)   1 only   D)   4 only   G)   1 and 4
B)   2 only   E)   1 and 2   H)   2 and 4 only
C)   3 only   F)   1 and 3   I)   3 and 4 only

Question 37:
Which of the following statements regarding respiration are correct?

1.   The mitochondria are the centres for both aerobic and anaerobic respiration.
2.   The cytoplasm is the main site of anaerobic respiration.
3.   For every two moles of glucose that is respired aerobically, 12 moles of CO_2 are liberated.
4.   Anaerobic respiration is more efficient than aerobic respiration.

A)   1 and 2   B)   1 and 4   C)   2 and 3   D)   2 and 4   E)   3 and 4

Question 38:
Which of the following statements are true?

1.   The nucleus contains the cell's chromosomes.
2.   The cytoplasm consists purely of water.
3.   The plasma membrane is a single phospholipid layer.
4.   The cell wall prevents plants cells from lysing due to osmotic pressure.

A)   1 and 2   C)   1, 3 and 4   E)   1, 2 and 4
B)   1 and 4   D)   1, 2 and 3   F)   2, 3 and 4

Question 39:
Which of the following statements are true about osmosis?

1.   If a medium is hypertonic relative to the cell cytoplasm, the cell will gain water through osmosis.
2.   If a medium is hypotonic relative to the cell cytoplasm, the cell will gain water through osmosis.
3.   If a medium is hypotonic relative to the cell cytoplasm, the cell will lose water through osmosis.
4.   If a medium is hypertonic relative to the cell cytoplasm, the cell will lose water through osmosis.
5.   The medium's tonicity has no impact on the movement of water.

A)   1 only   B)   2 only   C)   1 and 3   D)   2 and 4   E)   5 only

Question 40:
Which of the following statements are true about stem cells?

1. Stem cells have the ability to differentiate into other mature types of cells.
2. Stem cells are unable to maintain their undifferentiated state.
3. Stem cells can be classified as embryonic stem cells or adult stem cells.
4. Stem cells are only found in embryos.

A) 1 and 3
B) 3 and 4
C) 2 and 3
D) 1 and 2
E) 2 and 4

END OF SECTION

Section 3

Question 41:
Which of the following below is **NOT** an example of an oxidation reaction?

A) $Li^+ + H_2O \rightarrow Li^+ + OH^- + \frac{1}{2}H_2$
B) $N_2 \rightarrow 2N^+ + 2e^-$
C) $2CH_4 + 2O_2 \rightarrow 2CH_2O + 2H_2O$
D) $2N_2 + O_2 \rightarrow 2N_2O$
E) $I_2 + 2e^- \rightarrow 2I^-$
F) All of the above are oxidation reactions

Question 42:
Balance the following chemical equation. What is the value of **x**?

$w\ HIO_3 + 4FeI_2 + x\ HCl \rightarrow y\ FeCl_3 + z\ ICl + 15H_2O$

A) 4   C) 9   E) 22
B) 5   D) 15   F) 25

Question 43:
On analysis, an organic substance is found to contain 41.4% Carbon, 55.2% Oxygen and 3.45% Hydrogen by mass. Which of the following could be the chemical formula of this substance?

A) $C_3O_3H_6$ C) $C_4O_2H_4$ E) $C_4O_2H_8$
B) $C_3O_3H_{12}$ D) $C_4O_4H_4$ F) More information needed

Question 44:
$200\ cm^3$ of a $1.8\ moldm^{-3}$ solution of sodium nitrate ($NaNO_3$) is used in a chemical reaction. How many moles of sodium nitrate is this?

A) 0.09 mol   B) 0.36 mol   C) 9.00 mol   D) 36.0 mol   E) 360 mol

Question 45:
A is a group 3 element and B is a group 6 element. Which row best describes what happens to A when it reacts with B?

		Electrons are	Size of Atom
A)		Gained	Increases
B)		Gained	Decreases
C)		Gained	Unchanged
D)		Lost	Increases
E)		Lost	Decreases
F)		Lost	Unchanged

Question 46:
In relation to reactivity of elements in group 1 and 2, which of the following statements is correct?

1. Reactivity decreases as you go down group 1.
2. Reactivity increases as you go down group 2.
3. Group 1 metals are generally less reactive than group 2 metals.

A) Only 1   C) Only 3   E) 2 and 3
B) Only 2   D) 1 and 2   F) 1 and 3

Question 47:
What role do catalysts fulfil in an endothermic reaction?

A) They increase the temperature, causing the reaction to occur at a faster rate.
B) They decrease the temperature, causing the reaction to occur at a faster rate.
C) They reduce the energy of the reactants in order to trigger the reaction.
D) They reduce the activation energy of the reaction.
E) They increase the activation energy of the reaction.

Question 48:
Tritium H^3 is an isotope of Hydrogen. Why is tritium commonly referred to as 'heavy hydrogen'?

A) Because H^3 contains 3 protons making it heavier than H^1 that contains 1 proton.
B) Because H^3 contains 3 neutrons making it heavier than H^1 that contains 1 neutron.
C) Because H^3 contains 1 neutron and 2 protons making it heavier than H^1 that contains 1 neutron and 1 proton.
D) Because H^3 contains 1 proton and 2 neutrons making it heavier than H^1 that contains 1 proton.
E) Because H^3 contains 3 electrons making it heavier than H^1 that contains 1 electron.

Question 49:
Which of the following statements is correct?

A) At higher temperatures, gas molecules move at angles that cause them to collide with each other more frequently.
B) Gas molecules have lower energy after colliding with each other.
C) At higher temperatures, gas molecules attract each other resulting in more collisions.
D) The average kinetic energy of gas molecules is the same for all gases at the same temperature.
E) The momentum of gas molecules decreases as pressure increases.

Question 50:
In relation to redox reactions, which of the following statements are correct?

1. Oxidation describes the loss of electrons.
2. Reduction increases the electron density of an ion, atom or molecule.
3. Halogens are powerful reducing agents.

A) Only 1   C) Only 3   E) 2 and 3
B) Only 2   D) 1 and 2   F) 1 and 3

Question 51:
Which of the following are exothermic reactions?

1. Burning Magnesium in pure oxygen
2. The combustion of hydrogen
3. Aerobic respiration
4. Evaporation of water in the oceans
5. Reaction between a strong acid and a strong base

A) 1, 2 and 4   C) 1, 3 and 5   E) 1, 2, 3 and 5
B) 1, 2 and 5   D) 2, 3 and 4   F) 1, 2, 3, 4 and 5

Question 52:
Ethene reacts with oxygen to produce water and carbon dioxide. Which elements are oxidised/reduced?

A) Carbon is reduced, and oxygen is oxidised.
B) Hydrogen is reduced, and oxygen is oxidised.
C) Carbon is oxidised, and hydrogen is reduced.
D) Hydrogen is oxidised, and carbon is reduced.
E) Carbon is oxidised, and oxygen is reduced.
F) None of the above.

END OF SECTION

Section 4

Question 53:

The buoyancy force of an object is the produce of its volume, density and the gravitational constant, g. A boat weighing 600 kg with a density of 1000kgm^{-3} and hull volume of 950 litres is placed in a lake. What is the minimum mass that, if added to the boat, will cause it to sink? Use $g = 10 \text{ms}^{-1}$.

A) 3.55 kg

B) 35 kg

C) 350 kg

D) 355 kg

E) 3550 kg

F) None

Question 54:

Mr Khan fires a bullet at a speed of 310 ms^{-1} from a height of 1.93m parallel to the floor. Mr Weeks drops an identical bullet from the same height.

What is the time difference between the bullets first making contact with the floor? [Assume that there is negligible air resistance; g= 10 ms^{-2}]

A) 0 s

B) 0.2 s

C) 1.93 s

D) 2.1 s

E) More   information   needed

Question 55:

A 1.4kg fish swims through water at a constant speed of 2ms^{-1}. Resistive forces against the fish are 2N. Assuming $g = 10 \text{ms}^{-2}$, how much work does the fish do in one hour?

A) 7,200 J

B) 10,080 J

C) 14,400 J

D) 19,880 J

E) 22,500 J

F) More information needed

Question 56:

A crane is 40 m tall. The lifting arm is 5m long and the counterbalance arm is 2m long. The beam joining the two weighs 350kg, and is of uniform thickness. The lifting arm lifts a 2000 kg mass. What counterbalance mass is required to balance exactly around the centre point? Use $g = 10 \text{ ms}^{-2}$.

A) 4,220 kg

B) 4,820 kg

C) 5,013 kg

D) 5,263 kg

E) 10,525 kg

Question 57:

For Christmas, Mr James decorates his house with 20 strings of 150 bulbs each. Each 150-bulb string of lights is rated at 50 Watts. Mr James turns the lights on at 8pm and off at 6am each night. The lights are used for 20 days in total.

If 100 kJ of energy costs 2p, how much is the total cost Mr James has to pay?

A) £2160.00

B) £144.00

C) £14.40

D) £0.72

E) £0.24

Question 58:

Calculate the perimeter of a regular polygon each interior angle is 150° and each side is 15 cm.

A) 75 cm

B) 150 cm

C) 180 cm

D) 225 cm

E) 1,500 cm

F) More information needed.

Question 59:

The diagram shown below depicts an electrical circuit with multiple resistors, each with equal resistance, Z. The total resistance between A and B is 22 MΩ. Calculate the value of Z.

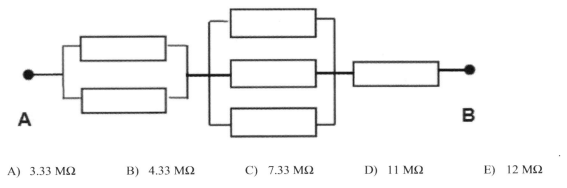

A) 3.33 MΩ B) 4.33 MΩ C) 7.33 MΩ D) 11 MΩ E) 12 MΩ

Question 60:

A cylindrical candle of diameter 4cm burns steadily at a rate of 1cm per hour. Assuming the candle is composed entirely of paraffin wax ($C_{24}H_{52}$) of density 900 kgm^{-3} and undergoes complete combustion, how much energy is transferred in 30 minutes? You may assume the molar combustion energy is 11,000 kJmol^{-1}, and that $\pi=3$.

A) 140,000J   C) 185,000J   E) 215,000J
B) 175,000J   D) 200,500J   F) 348,000J

END OF PAPER

MOCK PAPER F

Section 1

Question 1:
The first interstellar object to be detected passing through our solar system was discovered in 2017 by scientists in Hawaii; what was it named?

A) Oumuamua
B) Maui
C) Io
D) Hammurabi
E) Europa

Question 2:
In Greek mythology Zeus transformed into what animal to seduce Leda?

A) A goose
B) A Swan
C) A bull
D) A Mouse
E) A Horse

Question 3:
Which British monarch took over Hampton Court as his palace in 1529

A) James I
B) Edward I
C) Henry VII
D) Henry VIII
E) Edward VI

Question 4:
Anemometer is used to measure what?

A) Air pressure
B) Time
C) Windspeed
D) Depth
E) Altitude

Question 5:
The Taiping rebellion took place in which country?

A) Japan
B) Korea
C) Russia
D) China
E) Vietnam

Question 6:
Which scientist sailed on the Beagle to the Galapagos islands?

A) Charles Darwin
B) Gregor Mendel
C) Robert Brown
D) Rachel Carson
E) Alexander Fleming

Question 7:
Sir Isaac Newton and what other thinker both invented calculus at the same time?

A) Albert Einstein
B) Kurt Gödel
C) Baruch Spinoza
D) Gottfried Leibniz
E) Euclid

Question 8:
In 1819 the Peterloo massacre in Manchester occurred following a protest for what?

A) Tax relief
B) Parliamentary representation
C) An end to war
D) Lords reform
E) Free healthcare

Queston 9:
Which of these countries has never been in the European Union?

A) Switzerland
B) Spain
C) Austria
D) Sweden
E) Croatia

Question 10:
Which religion from Iran is the first known monotheistic religion?

A) Sikhism
B) Islam
C) Christianity
D) Judaism
E) Zoroastrianism

Question 11:
Which of these is not one of the official languages of India?

A) Hindi
B) Punjabi
C) Urdu
D) Bengali
E) Pashto

Question 12:

Which US president was in office during the Cuban missile crisis?

A) John F Kennedy
B) Lyndon B Johnson
C) George W Bush
D) Gerald Ford
E) Jimmy Carter

Question 13:

Every year, there are tens of thousands of motor crashes, causing a serious number of fatalities. Indeed, this represents the leading cause of death in the UK that is not a disease. In spite of this horrendous statistic, there are still thousands of uninsured drivers. The government is under moral obligation to clamp down on uninsured drivers, to reduce the incidence of such crashes. That they have not acted is arguably the most outrageous failing of the present government.

Which of the following is the best statement of a **flaw** in this passage?
A) It has made unsupported claims that the government's failure to act is morally outrageous.
B) It has not provided any evidence to support its claims that motor crashes are the leading cause of death in the UK outside of diseases.
C) Even if motor crashes were prevented, it would not save lives of people who die from other causes.
D) It has implied that lack of insurance is related to the incidence of motor crashes.
E) It has fabricated an obligation on the government's part to intervene and reduce the numbers of uninsured drivers.

Question 14:

Several years ago the Brazilian government held a referendum of the populace, to decide whether they should enact a law banning the ownership of guns. The Brazilian people voted strongly against this proposal. When asked why this had happened, one commentator said he believed the reason was that 90% of criminals who use guns to commit crimes buy their weapons on the black market, illegally. Thus, if Brazil were to ban the legal sale of guns, this would remove the ability of law-abiding citizens to purchase protection, whilst doing little to remove weapons from the hands of criminals.

Some commentators have pointed to this statistic, and claimed that the UK should also legalise guns, to allow citizens to protect themselves. However, in the UK the black market for weapons is not as widespread as in Brazil. Most people in the UK have little reason to fear gun attacks, and legalising the sale of guns would simply make it much easier for criminals to acquire weapons.

Which of the following best expresses the main conclusion of this passage?

A) The UK should not follow Brazil's lead on gun legislation.
B) Efforts to reduce gun ownership should focus on the black market.
C) Violent crime is a more pressing concern in Brazil than the UK.
D) Legalising the sale of guns in the UK would result in widespread ownership.
E) Criminals will always find a way to obtain firearms.

Question 15:

Hannah is buying tiles for her new bathroom. She wants to use the same tiles on the floor and all 4 walls and for all the walls to be completely tiled apart from the door. The bathroom is 2.4 metres high, 2 metres wide and 2 metres long, and the door is 2 metres high, 80cm wide and at the end of one of the 4 identical walls. The tiles she wants to use are 40cm x 40cm.

How many of these tiles does she need to tile the whole bathroom?

A) 110   B) 120   C) 135   D) 145   E) 15

Question 16:
Jane and Trevor are both travelling south, from York to London. Jane is driving, whilst Trevor is travelling by train. The speed limit on the roads between York and London is 70mph, whilst the train travels at 90mph. Thus, we should expect that Trevor will arrive first.

Which of the following would weaken this passage's conclusion?
A) The train takes a direct route, whilst the road from York to London goes through several major cities and zig-zags somewhat on its way down the country.
B) Trevor left before Jane.
C) Jane is a conscientious driver, who never exceeds the speed limit.
D) Trevor's train makes a lot of stops on the way, and spends several minutes at each stop waiting for new passengers to board.
E) Meanwhile, Raheem is making the same journey by plane, and will arrive before either Trevor or Jane.

Question 17:
ABC taxis charges a rate of 15p per minute, plus £4. XYZ taxis charges a rate of £4 plus 30p per mile. I live 6 miles from the station.

What would the taxi's average speed have to be on my journey home from the station for the two taxi firms to charge exactly the same fare?

A) 25   B) 30   C) 45   D) 55   E) 60

Question 18:
Adam's grandmother has sent him to the shop to buy bread rolls. Usually, bread rolls are 30p for a pack of 6 and so his grandmother has given him the exact amount to buy a certain number of bread rolls. However, today there is a special offer whereby if you buy 3 or more packs of rolls, the price per roll is reduced by 1p. He can now buy 1 more pack than before and get no change.
How many bread rolls was he originally supposed to buying?

A) 4   B) 5   C) 6   D) 24   E) 30

Question 19:

	Boys Absenteeism	Girls Absenteeism	Pupils on Roll	Average
Hazelwood Grammar	7%	Boys' School	300	7%
Heather Park Academy	5%	6%	1000	5.60%
Holland Wood Comprehensive	5%	6%	500	5.60%
Hurlington Academy	Girls' School		200	
Average		7%		

Some of the information is missing from the table above. What is the rate of girls' absenteeism at Hurlington Academy?

A) 6.5%   B) 7%   C) 9%   D) 11.5%   E) 13%

Question 20:

Harriet is a headmistress and she is making 400 information packs for the sixth form open evening. Each information pack needs to have 2 double sided sheets of A4 of general information about the school. She also needs to produce 50 A5 single sided sheets about each of the 30 A Level courses on offer. Single sided A5 costs £0.01 per sheet. Double sided costs twice as much as single sided. A4 printing costs 1.5 times as much as A5.

How much does she spend altogether on the printing?

A) £27   B) £31   C) £35   D) £39   E) £43

Question 21:

The pie chart shows the voting intentions of some constituents interviewed by a polling group, prior to an upcoming election.

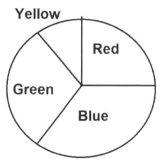

How many times more people said their intention was to vote for the red party than the yellow party?

A) 2   B) 3   C) 4   D) 5   E) 6

Question 22:

	Goals Scored	Goals Conceded
City	10	4
United	8	5
Rovers	1	10

The table above shows the goal scoring record of teams in a football tournament. Each team plays the other teams twice, once at home and once away. Here are the results of the first 4 matches:

➢ United 2 – 2 City   ➢ City 2 – 1 Rovers
➢ Rovers 0 – 3 City   ➢ Rovers 0 – 3 United

What were the results of the final two fixtures?

A) United 2 – 0 Rovers, City 0 – 0 United   D) United 1 – 0 Rovers, City 2 – 2 United
B) United 1 – 0 Rovers, City 1 – 1 United   E) United 2 – 0 Rovers, City 3 – 1 United
C) United 0 – 0 Rovers, City 2 – 1 United

END OF SECTION

Section 2

Question 23:
Why do cells undergo mitosis?

1. Asexual Reproduction
2. Sexual Reproduction
3. Growth of the human embryo
4. Replacement of dead cells

A) 1 only
B) 2 only
C) 3 only
D) 4 only

E) 2 and 3
F) 1, 2, and 3
G) 1, 3, and 4
H) 2, 3, and 4

Question 24:
In a healthy person, which one of the following has the highest blood pressure?

A) The vena cava
B) The systemic capillaries
C) The pulmonary artery

D) The pulmonary vein
E) The aorta
F) The coronary artery

The following information applies to questions 25 - 26:

Professor Huang accidentally touches a hot pan and her hand moves away in a reflex action. The diagram below shows a schematic of the reflex arc involved.

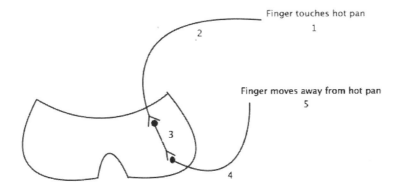

Question 25:
Which option correctly identifies the labels in the pathway?

	Muscle	Sensory Neurone	Receptor	Motor Neurone
A)	1	2	3	4
B)	2	3	1	5
C)	5	2	1	4
D)	1	4	5	2
E)	3	4	5	2
F)	4	2	1	3

Question 26:
Which one of the following statements is correct?

1. Information passes between 1 and 2 chemically.
2. Information passes between 2 and 3 electrically.
3. Information passes between 3 and 4 chemically.

A) 1 only
B) 2 only
C) 3 only

D) 1 and 2
E) 2 and 3
F) 1 and 3

G) All of the above
H) None of the above

Question 27:
For the following reaction, which of the statements below is true?

$$6CO_2 \text{ (g)} + 6H_2O \rightarrow C_6H_{12}O_6 + 6O_2 \text{ (g)}$$

A) Increasing the concentration of the products will increase the reaction rate.
B) Whether this reaction will proceed at room temperature is independent of the entropy.
C) The reaction rate can be monitored by measuring the volume of gas released.
D) This reaction represents aerobic respiration.
E) This reaction represents anaerobic respiration.

The following information applies to questions 28 - 29:

Duchenne muscular dystrophy (DMD) is inherited in an X-linked recessive pattern [transmitted on the X chromosome and requires the absence of normal X chromosomes to result in disease]. A man with DMD has two boys with a woman carrier.

Question 28:
What is the probability that both boys have DMD?

A) 100%
B) 75%

C) 50%
D) 25%

E) 12.5%
F) 0%

Question 29:
If the same couple had two more children, what is the probability that they are both girls with DMD?

A) 100%
B) 75%

C) 50%
D) 25%

E) 12.5%
F) 0%

Question 30:
Which of the following are **NOT** examples of natural selection?

1. Giraffes growing longer necks to eat taller plants.
2. Antibiotic resistance developed by certain strains of bacteria.
3. Pesticide resistance among locusts in farms.
4. Breeding of horses to make them run faster.

A) 1 only
B) 4 only

C) 1 and 3
D) 1 and 4

E) 2 and 4

Question 31:
Which row of the table is correct regarding the cell shown below?

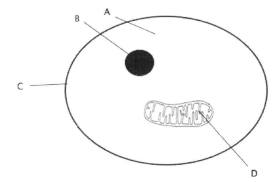

	Most Chemical Reactions occur here	Involved in Energy Release	Cell Type
A)	A	B	Animal
B)	A	B	Bacterial
C)	A	D	Animal
D)	B	D	Bacterial
E)	B	B	Animal
F)	B	A	Bacterial
G)	D	D	Animal
H)	D	B	Bacterial

Question 32:
Which of the following statements about white blood cells is correct?

1. They act by engulfing pathogens such as bacteria.
2. They are able to kill pathogens.
3. They transport carbon dioxide away from dying cells.

A) Only 1   D) 1 and 2   G) All
B) Only 2   E) 2 and 3   H) None
C) Only 3   F) 1 and 3

Question 33:
Which of the following statements are true?

1. Enzymes stabilise the transition state and therefore lower the activation energy.
2. Enzymes distort substrates in order to lower activation energy.
3. Enzymes decrease temperature to slow down reactions and lower the activation energy.
4. Enzymes provide alternative pathways for reactions to occur.

A) 1 only   C) 1 and 4   E) 3 and 4
B) 1 and 2   D) 2 and 4

Question 34:
Which of the following are examples of negative feedback?

1. Salivating whilst waiting for a meal.
2. Throwing a dart.

3. The regulation of blood pH.
4. The regulation of blood pressure.

A) 1 only
B) 1 and 2

C) 3 and 4
D) 2, 3, and 4

E) 1, 2, 3 and 4

Question 35:
Which of the following statements about the immune system are true?

1. White blood cells defend against bacterial and fungal infections.
2. White blood cells can temporarily disable but not kill pathogens.
3. White blood cells use antibodies to fight pathogens.
4. Antibodies are produced by bone marrow stem cells.

A) 1 and 3
B) 1 and 4

C) 2 and 3
D) 2 and 4

E) 1, 2, and 3
F) 1, 3, and 4

Question 36:
The cardiovascular system does **NOT**:

A) Deliver vital nutrients to peripheral cells.
B) Oxygenate blood and transports it to peripheral cells.
C) Act as a mode of transportation for hormones to reach their target organ.
D) Facilitate thermoregulation.
E) Respond to exercise by increasing cardiac output to exercising muscles.

Question 37:
Which of the following statements is correct?

A) Adrenaline can sometimes decrease heart rate.
B) Adrenaline is rarely released during flight or fight responses.
C) Adrenaline causes peripheral vasoconstriction.
D) Adrenaline only affects the cardiovascular system.
E) Adrenaline travels primarily in lymphatic vessels.
F) None of the above.

Question 38:
Which of the following statements is true?

A) Protein synthesis occurs solely in the nucleus.
B) Each amino acid is coded for by three DNA bases.
C) Each protein is coded for by three amino acids.
D) Red blood cells can create new proteins to prolong their lifespan.
E) Protein synthesis isn't necessary for mitosis to take place.
F) None of the above.

Question 39:

A solution of amylase and carbohydrate is present in a beaker, where the pH of the contents is 6.3. Assuming amylase is saturated, which of the following will increase the rate of production of the product?

1. Add sodium bicarbonate
2. Add carbohydrate
3. Add amylase
4. Increase the temperature to 100° C

A) 1 only
B) 2 only
C) 3 only
D) 4 only
E) 1 and 2
F) 1 and 3
G) 1, 2 and 3
H) 1, 3 and 4

Question 40:

Celestial Necrosis is a newly discovered autosomal recessive disorder. A female carrier and a male with the disease produce two boys. What is the probability that neither boy's genotype contains the celestial necrosis allele?

A) 100%
B) 75%
C) 50%
D) 25%
E) 0%

END OF SECTION

Section 3

Question 41:

Which of the following correctly describes the product of the reaction between hydrochloric acid and but-2-ene?

A) CH_3-CH_2-$C(Cl)H$-CH_3

B) CH_3-$C(Cl)$-CH_2-CH_3

C) $C(Cl)H_2$-CH_2-CH_2-CH_3

D) CH_3-CH_2-CH_2-$C(Cl)H_2$

E) None of the above.

Question 42:

The electrolysis of brine can be represented by the following equation: $2\ NaCl\ +\ 2\ X\ =\ 2\ Y\ +\ Z\ +\ Cl_2$
What are the correct formulae for X, Y and Z?

	X	Y	Z
A)	H_2O	H_2	O_2
B)	H_2O	NaOH	O_2
C)	H_2O	NaOH	H_2
D)	H_2	H_2O	O_2
E)	H_2	NaOH	O_2
F)	H_2	NaOH	H_2
G)	NaOH	H_2O	H_2
H)	NaOH	H_2O	O_2

Question 43:

An unknown element has two isotopes: ^{76}X and ^{78}X. $A_r = 76.5$. Which of the statements below are true of X?

1. ^{76}X is three times as abundant as ^{78}X.
2. ^{78}X is three times as abundant as ^{76}X.
3. ^{76}X is more stable than ^{78}X.

A)   1 only

B)   2 only

C)   3 only

D)   1 and 3

E)   2 and 3

F)   None of the above.

Question 44:

For the following reaction, which of the statements below is true?

$6CO_2$ (g) + $6H_2O$ → $C_6H_{12}O_6$ + $6O_2$ (g)

A) Increasing the concentration of the products will increase the reaction rate.

B) Whether this reaction will proceed at room temperature is independent of the entropy.

C) The reaction rate can be monitored by measuring the volume of gas released.

D) This reaction represents aerobic respiration.

E) This reaction represents anaerobic respiration.

Question 45:
Which of the following are true about the formation of polymers?

1. They are formed from saturated molecules.
2. Water is released when polymers form.
3. Polymers only form linear molecules.

A) Only 1   D) 1 and 2   G) All of the above.
B) Only 2   E) 1 and 3   H) None of the above.
C) Only 3   F) 2 and 3

Question 46:
In the reaction between Zinc and Copper (II) sulphate which elements act as oxidising + reducing agents?

A) Zinc is the reducing agent while sulfur is the oxidizing agent.
B) Zinc is the reducing agent while copper in $CuSO_4$ is the oxidizing agent.
C) Copper is the reducing agent while zinc is the oxidizing agent.
D) Oxygen is the reducing agent while copper in $CuSO_4$ is the oxidizing agent.
E) Sulfur is the reducing agent while oxygen is the oxidizing agent.
F) None of the above.

Question 47:
Which of the following statements is true?

A) Acids are compounds that act as proton acceptors in aqueous solution.
B) Acids only exist in a liquid state.
C) Strong acids are partially ionized in a solution.
D) Weak acids generally have a pH or 6 - 7.
E) The reaction between a weak and strong acid produces water and salt.

Question 48:
An unknown element, Z, has 3 isotopes: Z^5, Z^6 and Z^8. Given that the atomic mass of Z is 7, and the relative abundance of Z^5 is 20%, which of the following statements are correct?

1. Z^5 and Z^6 are present in the same abundance.
2. Z^8 is the most abundant of the isotopes.
3. Z^8 is more abundant than Z^5 and Z^6 combined

A) 1 only   E) 2 and 3 only
B) 2 only   F) 1 and 3 only
C) 3 only   G) 1, 2 and 3
D) 1 and 2 only   H) None of the statements are correct.

Question 49:
Which of following best describes the products when an acid reacts with a metal that is more reactive than hydrogen?

A) Salt and hydrogen   D) A weak acid and a weak base
B) Salt and ammonia   E) A strong acid and a strong base
C) Salt and water   F) No reaction would occur.

Question 50:

Choose the option which balances the following equation:

a $FeSO_4$ + **b** $K_2Cr_2O_7$ + **c** H_2SO_4 → **d** $(Fe)_2(SO_4)_3$ + **e** $Cr_2(SO_4)_3$ + **f** K_2SO_4 + **g** H_2O

	a	b	c	d	e	f	g
A	6	1	8	3	1	1	7
B	6	1	7	3	1	1	7
C	2	1	6	2	1	1	6
D	12	1	14	4	1	1	14
E	4	1	12	4	1	1	12
F	8	1	8	4	2	1	8

Question 51:

Which of the following statements is correct?

A) Matter consists of atoms that have a net electrical charge.
B) Atoms and ions of the same element have different numbers of protons and electrons but the same number of neutrons.
C) Over 80% of an atom's mass is provided by protons.
D) Atoms of the same element that have different numbers of neutrons react at significantly different rates.
E) Protons in the nucleus of atoms repel each other as they are positively charged.
F) None of the above.

Question 52:

Which of the following statements is correct?

A) The noble gasses are chemically inert and therefore useless to man.
B) All the noble gasses have a full outer electron shell.
C) The majority of noble gasses are brightly coloured.
D) The boiling point of the noble gasses decreases as you progress down the group.
E) Neon is the most abundant noble gas.

END OF SECTION

Section 4

Question 53:

A ball of radius 2 m and density 3 kg/m³ is released from the top of a frictionless ramp of height 20m and rolls down. What is its speed at the bottom? Take $\pi = 3$ and $g = 10\text{m}^{-2}$.

A) 1 ms⁻¹

B) 4 ms⁻¹

C) 7 ms⁻¹

D) 9 ms⁻¹

E) 14 ms⁻¹

F) 20 ms⁻¹

Question 54:

Which of the following statements is true regarding waves?

A) Waves can transfer mass in the direction of propagation.

B) All waves have the same energy.

C) All light waves have the same energy.

D) Waves can interfere with each other.

E) None of the above.

Question 55:

Rearrange $\frac{(7x+10)}{(9x+5)} = 3z^2 + 2$, to make x the subject.

A) $x = \frac{15\,z^2}{7 - 9(3z^2+2)}$

B) $x = \frac{15\,z^2}{7 + 9(3z^2+2)}$

C) $x = -\frac{15\,z^2}{7 - 9(3z^2+2)}$

D) $x = -\frac{15\,z^2}{7 + 9(3z^2+2)}$

E) $x = -\frac{15\,z^2}{7 + 3(3z^2+2)}$

F) $x = \frac{15\,z^2}{7 + 3(3z^2+2)}$

Question 56:

Element $^{188}_{90}X$ decays into two equal daughter nuclei after a single alpha decay and the release of gamma radiation. What is the daughter element?

A) $^{91}_{45}D$

B) $^{92}_{44}D$

C) $^{184}_{88}D$

D) $^{186}_{90}D$

E) $^{186}_{45}D$

Question 57:

The diagram below shows a series of identical sports fields:

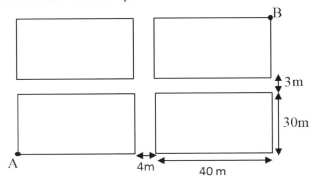

Calculate the shortest distance between points A and B.

A) 100 m

B) 105 m

C) 146 m

D) 148 m

E) 154 m

F) None of the above.

Question 58:

Calculate $\dfrac{1.25 \times 10^{10} + 1.25 \times 10^9}{2.5 \times 10^8}$

A) 0

B) 1

C) 55

D) 110

E) 1.25×10^8

F) 5.5×10^7

G) 5.5×10^8

Question 59:

Solve $y = 2x - 1$ and $y = x^2 - 1$ for x and y.

A) (0, -1) and (2, 3)

B) (1, -1) and (2, 2)

C) (1, 4) and (3, 2)

D) (2, -3) and (4, 5)

E) (3, -1) and (3, 1)

F) (4, -2) and (-2, 4)

Question 60:

Tim stands at the waterfront and holds a 30 cm ruler horizontally at eye level one metre in front of him. It lines up so it appears to be exactly the same length as a cruise ship 1 km out to sea. How long is the cruise ship?

A) 299.7 m

B) 300.0 m

C) 333.3 m

D) 29,970 m

E) 30,000 m

END OF PAPER

MOCK PAPER G

Section 1

Question 1:
The Qabbalah is a series of mystical teachings derived from which religion?

A) Christianity
B) Judaism
C) Islam
D) Buddhism
E) Sikhism

Question 2:
The eruption of Vesuvius destroyed what Roman city?

A) Naples
B) Pompeii
C) Florence
D) Herculaneum
E) Paestum

Question 3:
Guernica is a painting by Pablo Picasso completed in 1937 commemorating what event in the town's history?

A) Bombing
B) Tsunami
C) Earthquake
D) Festival
E) Evacuation

Question 4:
Dinosaur is Greek for what?

A) Large reptile
B) Scaly bird
C) Terrible lizard
D) Frightening creature
E) Tall snake

Question 5:
Clio, Erato and Thalia are three of the nine what, who inspired artists in Greek myth?

A) Nymphs
B) Satyrs
C) Muses
D) Gremlins
E) Sages

Question 6:
What world leader was placed under house arrest in 2017 after 37 years of rule?

A) Xi Jingping
B) Robert Mugabe
C) Hassan Rouhani
D) Abdulla Aripov
E) Rodrigo Duterte

Question 7:

Martin Luther famously nailed his 95 theses to the door of a church in protest of what institution?

A) The Monarchy
B) Parliament
C) The Catholic Church
D) The Eastern Orthodox Church
E) Guilds

Question 8:

In 1948 the UN published a chart of 30 articles protecting what?

A) The Environment
B) Human Rights
C) Birds
D) National Sovereignty
E) Religion

Question 9:

Galileo and Copernicus both argued for a helio-centric model of the universe replacing who's commonly used model?

A) Aristotle
B) Plato
C) Ptolemy
D) Cicero
E) Seneca

Question 10:

The Higgs Boson was discovered by the LHC at CERN, what does LHC stand for?

A) Large Hadron collider
B) Large Helium Container
C) Large Higgs Collector
D) Linear hydrogen Container
E) Little Higgs Collider

Question 11:

The Uffizi gallery in Florence is famous for the world largest collection of what?

A) Roman artefacts
B) Historical Weapons
C) Impressionist paintings
D) Renaissance paintings
E) Renaissance sculpture

Question 12:

Seven people died in the Challenger disaster of 1986, what was the Challenger?

A) A ship
B) A helicopter
C) A space shuttle
D) A truck
E) A zeppelin

Question 13:

Irish Folk Band, the Willow, have recently signed a contract with a new manager, and are organising a new musical tour. They and their manager are discussing which country would be best to organise their tour in. The lead singer of the willow would like to organise a tour in Germany, which has a rich history of folk music. However, the new manager finds that ticket sales for folk music concerts in Germany have been steadily declining for several years, whilst France has recently seen a significant increase in ticket sales for folk music concerts. The manager says that this means the group's ticket sales would be higher if they organise a tour in France, than if they organise one in Germany.

Which of the following is an assumption that the manager has made?

A) The band should prioritise profits and organise a tour in the most profitable country possible.
B) The band should not embark upon a new tour and should instead focus on record sales.
C) The decrease of ticket sales in Germany and the increase in France means that the band will sell fewer tickets in Germany than in France.
D) There will not be other countries which are even more profitable than France to organise the tour in.
E) Folk music is popular in France.

Question 14:

John is a train enthusiast, who has been studying the directions in which trains travel after departing from various London Stations. He finds that Trains departing from King's Cross station in London head North on the East Coast Mainline, and travel to Edinburgh. Trains departing from Waterloo Station head West on the Southwest Mainline and travel to Plymouth. Trains departing from Victoria Station head South and travel to Kent. John surmises that presently, in order to travel on a train from London to Edinburgh, he must get on at King's Cross Station.

Which of the following is an assumption that John has made?

A) The East Coast mainline has the fastest trains.
B) It would not be quicker to take a train from Waterloo to Southampton Airport, then travel to Edinburgh on an Aeroplane.
C) Rail lines will not be built that will allow trains to travel from Waterloo Station or Victoria Station to Edinburgh.
D) King's Cross trains do not have any other destinations other than Edinburgh.
E) There are no other train stations in London from which trains may travel to Edinburgh.

Question 15:

I write my 4 digit pin number down in a coded format, by multiplying the first and second number together, dividing by the third number than subtracting the fourth number. If my code is 3, which of these could my pin number be?

A) 3461   B) 9864   C) 5423   D) 7848   E) 6849

Question 16:

Rental yield for buy to let properties is calculated by dividing the potential rent per year paid for a house by the amount it cost to buy the house and get it in a rentable condition. Tina is considering 5 houses as possible buy to let investments. House A is in good condition and could be rented as it is for £700 a month, and costs £168,000 to buy. House B is also in good condition but is a student house, so Tina would need to buy furniture for it. The house would cost £190,000 to buy and £10,000 to furnish but could be rented for 40 weeks of the year to 4 students at a rent of £125 a week each. House C needs a lot of work doing. It costs £100,000 but would need £44,000 of renovations and would rent for £600 a month. House D costs £200,000 and would need £40,000 of renovations and would rent out for £2000 a month. House E costs £80,000 and would need £20,000 of renovations and could be rented out for £200 a week.

Which house has the highest rental yield?

A) A   B) B   C) C   D) D   E) E

Question 17:

Summer and Shaniqua are playing a game of "noughts and crosses". Each player is assigned either "noughts" (O) or "crosses" (X) and they take it in turns to choose an empty box of the 3x3 grid to put their symbol in. The winner is the first person to get a line of 3 of their symbol in any direction in the grid (vertically, horizontally or diagonally). Summer starts the game. The current position is shown below:

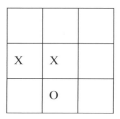

Assuming Shaniqua now plays her symbol in the square which will stop Summer being able to win the game straight away, Summer should play in either of which 2 boxes to ensure she is able to win the game on the next turn no matter what Shaniqua does?

1	2	3
		4
6		5

A) 1 and 3   B) 1 and 5   C) 1 and 6   D) 2 and 4   E) 3 and 5

Question 18:

A packaging company wishes to make cardboard boxes by taking a flat 1.2 m by 1.2 m square piece of cardboard, cutting square sections out of each corner as shown by the picture below and folding up the sections remaining on each side to make a box. The company experiments with different size boxes by cutting differently sized squares from the corners each time. It makes a box with 10 cm by 10 cm squares cut out of each corner, a box with 20 cm by 20 cm squares cut out of each corner and so on up to one with 50 cm by 50 cm squares cut out of each corner.

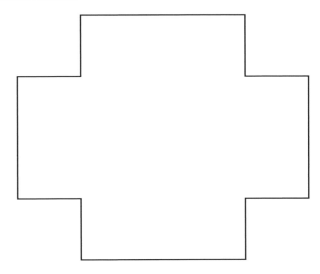

Which side length cut out would result in a box with the largest volume?

A) 10 cm   B) 20 cm   C) 30 cm   D) 40 cm   E) 50 cm

Question 19:

The aeroplane was a marvel of modern engineering when it was first developed in the early 20th Century, and was testament to human ingenuity. Throughout the 20th Century, the aeroplane allowed humans to travel more freely and widely than ever before, and allowed people to see and appreciate the stunning natural beauty the world has to offer. However, Aeroplanes also produce lots of pollution, such as Carbon Dioxide and Sulphur Oxide. High levels of Carbon Dioxide in the atmosphere are currently causing global warming, which is destroying or damaging many natural environments throughout the world.

Therefore it is clear that the aeroplane, which once offered such opportunity to appreciate the world's natural beauty, has been largely responsible for damage to various natural environments throughout the world. We must now seek to curb air traffic in order to save the world's remaining natural environments.

Which of the following is the best statement of a flaw in this argument?

A) It assumes that aeroplanes are a major reason for the high levels of Carbon Dioxide in the atmosphere which are currently causing global warming.
B) It assumes that aeroplanes offer greater opportunity to appreciate the world's natural environments.
C) It assumes that high levels of Carbon Dioxide are responsible for global warming.
D) It does not consider the effects of Sulphur Dioxide pollution released by aeroplanes.
E) It implies that we should take action to prevent damage to the world's natural environments.

Question 20:

There has recently been a new election in the UK, and the new government is pondering what policy to adopt on the railway system in the UK. The Finance Minister argues that the best policy is to have an entirely privatised railway system, which will encourage different train companies to be competitive, and try and attract customers by providing the best service at the lowest price, thus driving down costs and increasing quality for customers. However, the Transport Minister argues that this is a short-sighted policy. She argues that privatised companies will only run services on the most profitable lines, where there are lots of passengers.

Under this system, train companies may not choose to run many services to rural areas. This will lead to rural communities being cut off, with a consequent lack of opportunities for people in these communities. She argues that public funding should be put towards rail services in order to ensure that people in rural communities are adequately served by rail services.

Which of the following, if true, would most strengthen the Transport Minister's argument?

A) The Transport Minister has ultimate power over railway policy, and she can overrule the Chancellor if she sees fit.
B) Many train services to rural communities currently have low passenger numbers, and are unlikely to be profitable.
C) French rail services receive high level of public funding, and users of these services enjoy good quality and low prices.
D) American railway services are privatised with no public funding, and yet rural communities in America are well served by railway services.
E) The Prime Minister agrees with the Transport Minister's line of argument. He sympathises with rural communities and does not believe in a privatised rail system.

Question 21:

Global warming is widely presented in modern society as a cause for significant concern. One particular area often thought to be at risk is the Ice caps of the North and South Poles, which are often presented to be at risk of melting due to increased temperature. Environmentalist groups often campaign for energy consumption to be reduced, thus reducing CO_2 emissions, the leading cause of global warming. However, recent research shows that the North and South Poles are actually becoming cooler, not warmer, thanks to mysterious and unexplained weather patterns. Clearly, high energy consumption is not contributing to damage to the Polar Ice caps.

Which of the following statements can be reliably inferred from this argument?

A) There is no point in reducing energy consumption for environmental reasons.
B) Reducing energy consumption will not reduce CO_2 emissions.
C) We should trust the recent research stating that the North and South poles are becoming cooler.
D) Reducing energy consumption will not contribute to saving the polar ice caps.
E) We should not be concerned about damage to the Polar Ice caps.

Question 22:
Penicillin is one of the major success stories of modern medicine. Since its discovery in 1928, it has grown to become a crucial foundation of medicine, saving countless lives and introducing the age of antibiotics. Alexander Fleming is today given most of the credit for introducing and developing antibiotics, but in fact Fleming played a relatively minor role. Fleming initially discovered Penicillin, but was unable to demonstrate its clinical effectiveness, or discern ways of reliably and consistently producing it. 2 other scientists called Howard Florey and Ernst Chain were actually responsible for developing Penicillin to the point where it could be reliably produced and used in medicine, to treat infections in patients. Clearly, the credit for the wonders worked by Penicillin should not go to Fleming, but to Florey and Chain.

Which of the following best illustrates the main conclusion of this argument?

A) Fleming was unable to develop penicillin to the point of being a viable medical treatment.
B) The credit for Penicillin's effects on medicine should go to Ernst Chain and Howard Florey, not to Alexander Fleming.
C) Without Chain and Florey, Penicillin would not have been developed into a viable treatment.
D) Alexander Fleming only played a small role in the process of Penicillin becoming a feature of modern medicine.
E) Alexander Fleming is not given enough credit for his role in the development of penicillin.

END OF SECTION

Section 2

Question 23:
Which of the following statements are true?

1. Natural selection always favours organisms that are faster or stronger.
2. Genetic variation leads to different adaptations to the environment.
3. Variation is purely due to genetics.

A) Only 1
B) Only 2
C) Only 3

D) 1 and 2
E) 2 and 3
F) 1 and 3

G) All of the above.
H) None of the above.

The following information applies to questions 24 – 25:

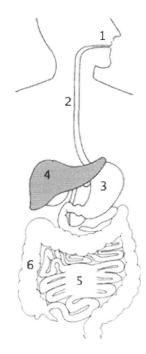

Question 24:
Which of the following numbers indicate where amylase functions?

A) 1 only
B) only
C) 1 and 3

D) 1 and 5
E) 2 and 4
F) 3 and 4

G) 5 and 6

Question 25:
In which of the following does the majority of chemical digestion occur?

A) 1
B) 2
C) 3

D) 4
E) 5
F) 6

G) None of the above.

The following information applies to questions 26-27:

The diagram below shows the genetic inheritance of colour-blindness, which is inherited in a sex-linked recessive manner [transmitted on the X chromosome and requires the absence of normal X chromosomes to result in disease]. X^B is the normal allele and X^b is the colour-blind allele.

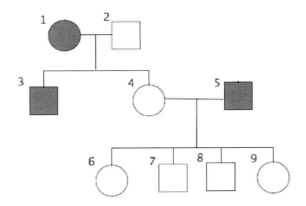

Question 26:

What is the genotype of the individual marked 4?

A) $X^B X^b$ B) $X^B X^B$ C) $X^b X^b$ D) $X^B Y$ E) $X^b Y$

Question 27:

If 8 were to reproduce with a heterozygote female, what is the probability of producing a colour-blind boy?

A) 100%   C) 50%   E) 12.5%

B) 75%   D) 25%   F) 0%

Question 28:

Which of the following correctly describes the passage of urine through the body?

	1st	2nd	3rd	4th
A	Kidney	Ureter	Bladder	Urethra
B	Kidney	Urethra	Bladder	Ureter
C	Urethra	Bladder	Ureter	Kidney
D	Ureter	Kidney	Bladder	Urethra

The following information applies to questions 29 – 30:

In pea plants, colour and stem length are inherited in an autosomal manner. The allele for yellow colour, Y, is dominant to the allele for green colour, y. Furthermore, the allele for tall stem length, T, is dominant to short stem length, t.

When a pea plant of unknown genotype is crossed with a green short-stemmed pea plant, the progeny are 25% yellow + tall-stemmed plants, 25% yellow + short-stemmed plants, 25% green + tall-stemmed plants and 25% green + short-stemmed plants.

Question 29:

What is the genotype of the unknown pea plant?

A) Yytt
B) YyTt

C) YyTT
D) yyTt

E) yyTT
F) yytt

Question 30:

Taking both colour and height into account, how many different combinations of genotypes and phenotypes are possible?

A) 6 genotypes and 3 phenotypes
B) 8 genotypes and 3 phenotypes
C) 8 genotypes and 4 phenotypes
D) 9 genotypes and 4 phenotypes
E) 9 genotypes and 3 phenotypes
F) 10 genotypes and 3 phenotypes

Question 31:

What is the **MOST** important reason for each cell in the human body to have an adequate blood supply?

A) To allow protein synthesis.
B) To receive essential minerals and vitamins for life.
C) To kill invading bacteria.
D) To allow aerobic respiration to take place.
E) To maintain an optimum cellular temperature.
F) To maintain an optimum cellular pH.

Question 32:

Which of the following statements are true?

1. Increasing levels of insulin cause a decrease in blood glucose levels.
2. Increasing levels of glycogen cause an increase in blood glucose levels.
3. Increasing levels of adrenaline decrease the heart rate.

A) 1 only
B) 2 only

C) 3 only
D) 1 and 2

E) 2 and 3
F) 1 and 3

G) 1, 2 and 3

Question 33:

Which of the following rows is correct?

	Oxygenated Blood		Deoxygenated Blood	
A.	Left atrium	Left ventricle	Right atrium	Right ventricle
B.	Left atrium	Right atrium	Left ventricle	Right ventricle
C.	Left atrium	Right ventricle	Right atrium	Right ventricle
D.	Right atrium	Right ventricle	Left atrium	Left ventricle
E.	Left ventricle	Right atrium	Left atrium	Right ventricle

Questions 34-36 are based on the following information:
The pedigree below shows the inheritance of a newly discovered disease that affects connective tissue called Nafram syndrome. Individual 1 is a normal homozygote.

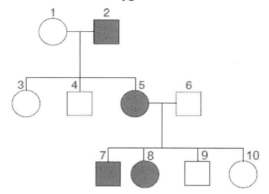

Question 34:
What is the inheritance of Nafram syndrome?

A) Autosomal dominant
B) Autosomal recessive
C) X-linked dominant
D) X-linked recessive
E) Co-dominant

Question 35:
Which individuals must be heterozygous for Nafram syndrome?

A) 1 and 2
B) 8 and 9
C) 2 and 5
D) 5 and 6
E) 6 and 8
F) 6 and 10

Question 36:
Taking N to denote a diseased allele and n to denote a normal allele, which of the following are **NOT** possible genotypes for 6's parents?

1. NN x NN
2. NN x Nn
3. Nn x nn
4. Nn x Nn
5. nn x nn

A) 1 and 2
B) 1 and 3
C) 2 and 3
D) 2 and 5
E) 3 and 4
F) 4 and 5

Question 37:
Which among the following has no endocrine function?

A) The thyroid
B) The ovary
C) The pancreas
D) The adrenal gland
E) The testes
F) None of the above.

Question 38:
Which of the following best describes the passage of blood from the body, through the heart, back to the body?

A) Aorta → Left Ventricle → Left Atrium → Inferior Vena Cava → Right Atrium → Right Ventricle → Lungs
B) Inferior vena cava → Left Atrium → Left Ventricle → Lungs → Right Atrium → Right Ventricle → Aorta
C) Inferior vena cava → Right Ventricle → Right Atrium → Lungs → Left Atrium → Left Ventricle → Aorta
D) Aorta → Left Atrium → Left Ventricle → Lungs → Right Atrium → Right Ventricle → Inferior Vena Cava
E) Right Atrium → Left Atrium → Inferior vena cava → Lungs → Left Atrium → Right Ventricle → Aorta
F) None of the above.

Question 39:
Which of the following best describes the events during inspiration?

	Intrathoracic Pressure	Intercostal Muscles	Diaphragm
A	Increases	Contract	Contracts
B	Increases	Relax	Contracts
C	Increases	Contract	Relaxes
D	Increases	Relax	Relaxes
E	Decreases	Contract	Contracts
F	Decreases	Relax	Contracts
G	Decreases	Contract	Relaxes
H	Decreases	Relax	Relaxes

Question 40:
Which row of the table below describes what happens when external temperature decreases?

	Temperature Change Detected by	Sweat Gland Secretion	Cutaneous Blood Flow
A	Hypothalamus	Increases	Increases
B	Hypothalamus	Increases	Decreases
C	Hypothalamus	Decreases	Increases
D	Hypothalamus	Decreases	Decreases
E	Cerebral Cortex	Increases	Increases
F	Cerebral Cortex	Increases	Decreases
G	Cerebral Cortex	Decreases	Increases
H	Cerebral Cortex	Decreases	Decreases

END OF SECTION

Section 3

Question 41:

Which of the following statements are true about the electrolysis of brine?

1. It describes the reduction of 2 chloride ions to Cl_2.
2. The amount of NaOH produced increases in proportion with the amount of NaCl present in solution, provided there is enough H_2 present to dissolve the NaCl.
3. The redox reaction of the electrolysis of brine results in the production of dissolved NaOH, which is a strong acid.

A) Only 1   E) 1 and 3
B) Only 2   F) 2 and 3
C) Only 3   G) All of the above.
D) 1 and 2   H) None of the above.

Question 42:

Which of the following correctly describes the product of the reaction between propene and hydrofluoric acid (HF)?

A) $C(F)H_3-CH_2-CH_3$ D) $CH_3-C(F)H_2-CH_3$
B) $CH_3-C(F)H-CH_3$ E) None of the above.
C) $CH_3-C(F)H_2-CH_2$

Question 43:

Which of the following are true about the reaction between alkenes and hydrogen halides?

1. The product formed is fully saturated.
2. The hydrogen halide binds at the alkene's saturated double bond.
3. The hydrogen halide forms ionic bonds with the alkene.

A) Only 1   E) 2 and 3
B) Only 2   F) 1 and 3
C) Only 3   G) All of the above.
D) 1 and 2   H) None of the above.

Question 44:

For the following reaction, which of the statements below are true?

$$N_{2(g)} + 3\ H_{2(g)} \rightleftharpoons 2\ NH_{3(g)}$$

1. Increasing pressure will cause the equilibrium to shift to the right.
2. Increasing pressure will form more ammonia gas.
3. Increasing the concentration of N_2 will create more ammonia.

A) 1 only   E) 2 and 3
B) 2 only   F) All of the above.
C) 3 only   G) None of the above.
D) 1 and 2

Question 45:

When sodium and chlorine react to form salt, which of the following best represents the bonding and electron configurations of the products and reactants?

	Sodium (s)		Chlorine (g)		Salt (s)	
	Intra-element bond	Element electron configuration	Intra-element bond	Element electron configuration	Compound bond	Compound electron configuration
A)	Ionic	2, 8, 1	Covalent	2, 8, 8, 1	Ionic	2, 8, 1 : 2, 8, 8, 1
B)	Metallic	2, 7	Covalent	2, 8, 1	Ionic	2, 8 : 2, 8
C)	Covalent	2, 8, 2	Ionic	2, 8, 8	Covalent	2, 8 : 2, 8, 8
D)	Ionic	2, 7	Ionic	2, 8, 8, 7	Covalent	2, 7 : 2, 8, 8, 7
E)	Metallic	2, 8, 1	Covalent	2, 8, 7	Ionic	2, 8 : 2, 8, 8

Question 46:

Which of the following correctly describes the product of the polymerisation of chloroethene molecules?

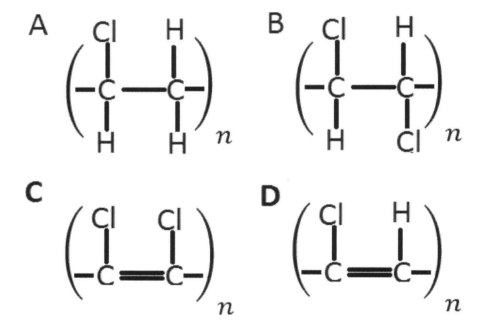

Question 47:

An organic molecule contains 70.6% Carbon, 5.9% Hydrogen and 23.5% Oxygen. It has a molecular mass of 136. What is its chemical formula?

A. C_4H_4O
B. C_5H_4O
C. $C_8H_8O_2$
D. $C_{10}H_8O_2$
E. C_2H_2O

Question 48:

In relation to alkenes, which of the following statements is correct?

1. They all contain double bonds.
2. They can all be reduced to alkanes.
3. Aromatic compounds are also alkenes as they contain double bonds.

A. Only 1
B. Only 2
C. Only 3

D. 1 and 2
E. 2 and 3
F. 1 and 3

G. All of the above.
H. None of the above.

Question 49:

Which of the following statements regarding transition metals is correct?

A. Transition metals form ions that have multiple colours.
B. Transition metals usually form covalent bonds.
C. Transition metals cannot be used as catalysts as they are too reactive.
D. Transition metals are poor conductors of electricity.
E. Transition metals are frequently referred to as f-block elements.

Question 50:

Chlorine is made up of two isotopes, Cl^{35} (atomic mass 34.969) and Cl^{37} (atomic mass 36.966). Given that the atomic mass of chlorine is 35.453, which of the following statements is correct?
A. Cl^{35} is about 3 times more abundant than Cl^{37}.
B. Cl^{35} is about 10 times more abundant than Cl^{37}.
C. Cl^{37} is about 3 times more abundant than Cl^{35}.
D. Cl^{37} is about 10 times more abundant than Cl^{35}.
E. Both isotopes are equally abundant.

Question 51:

20 g of impure Na^{23} reacts completely with excess water to produce 8,000 cm³ of hydrogen gas under standard conditions. What is the percentage purity of sodium?
[Under standard conditions 1 mole of gas occupies 24 dm³]

A. 88.0%   B. 76.5%   C. 66.0%   D. 38.0%   E. 15.3%

Question 52:
Choose the option which balances the following reaction:

aS + bHNO₃ → cH₂SO₄ + dNO₂ + eH₂O

	a	b	c	d	e
A	3	5	3	5	1
B	1	6	1	6	2
C	6	14	6	14	2
D	2	4	2	4	4
E	2	3	2	3	2
F	4	4	4	4	2

END OF SECTION

Section 4

Question 53:
Which of the following statements is **FALSE**?

A) A nuclear power plant may have an accident if free neutrons in a fuel rod aren't captured.
B) Humans cannot currently harness the energy from nuclear fusion.
C) Uncontrolled nuclear fission leads to a large explosion.
D) Mass is conserved during nuclear explosions caused by nuclear bombs.
E) Nuclear fusion produces much more energy than nuclear fission.

Question 54:
Rearrange the following to make m the subject.

$$T = 4\pi\sqrt{\frac{(M + 3m)l}{3(M + 2m)g}}$$

A) $m = \frac{16\pi^2 lM - 3gMT^2}{48\pi^2 l - 6gT^2}$

C) $m = \frac{3gMT^2 - 16\pi^2 lM}{6gT^2 - 48\pi^2 l}$

E) $m = \left(\frac{16\pi^2 lM - 3gMT^2}{6gT^2 - 48\pi^2 l}\right)^2$

B) $m = \frac{16\pi^2 lM - 3gMT^2}{6gT^2 - 48\pi^2 l}$

D) $m = \frac{4\pi^2 lM - 3gMT^2}{6gT^2 - 16\pi^2 l}$

Question 55:
The mean of a set of 11 numbers is 6. Two numbers are removed and the mean is now 5. Which of the following is not a possible combination of removed numbers?

A. 1 and 20   B. 6 and 9   C. 10 and 11   D. 15 and 6   E. 19 and 2

Question 56:
Which will have a greater current, a circuit with two identical resistors in series or one with the same two resistors in parallel?

A) Series will have greater current than parallel.   C) Same current in both.
B) Parallel will have greater current than series.   D) It depends on the battery.

Question 57:
Evaluate: $\frac{3.4 \times 10^{11} + 3.4 \times 10^{10}}{6.8 \times 10^{12}}$

A) 5.5×10^{-12} C) 5.5×10^1 E) 5.5×10^{10}
B) 5.5×10^{-2} D) 5.5×10^2 F) 5.5×10^{12}

Question 58:

Find the values of angles b and c.

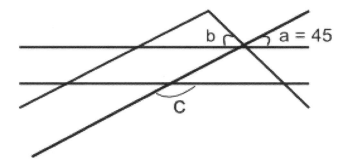

A) 45° and 135°

B) 45° and 130°

C) 50° and 135°

D) 55° and 130°

E) More information needed.

Question 59:

Which of the following statements is true regarding electrolysis?

A) Using an AC-current is most effective.

B) Using a DC-current is most effective.

C) An AC-current causes cations to gather at the cathode.

D) A DC-current would plate the anode in copper from a copper sulphate solution.

E) No current is used in electrolysis.

Question 60:

Evaluate the following expression:

$$\left(\left(\tfrac{6}{8} \times \tfrac{7}{3}\right) \div \left(\tfrac{7}{5} \times \tfrac{2}{6}\right)\right) \times 0.40 \times 15\% \times 5\% \times \pi \times \left(\sqrt{e^2}\right) \times 0.20 \times (e\pi)^{-1}$$

A) $\dfrac{4}{55}$

B) $\dfrac{8}{770}$

C) $\dfrac{9}{4,000}$

D) $\dfrac{8}{54,321}$

E) $\dfrac{9}{67,800}$

END OF PAPER

MOCK PAPER H

Section 1

Question 1:
What building in Spain was started in 1882, and has yet to be completed?

A) The Alhambra
B) The Güell Park
C) The Casa Mila
D) The Sagrada Familia
E) The Guggenheim

Question 2:
Pslams, Proverbs and Ecclesiastes are collectively known as the what books of the Bible?

A) Minor Prophets
B) Major Prophets
C) Laws
D) Songs and Wisdom Literature
E) History

Question 3:
Where did the Mau Mau uprising against the British in the 1950's take place?

A) India
B) South Africa
C) Kenya
D) Jamaica
E) Zimbabwe

Question 4:
'Man is born free, but everywhere he is in chains' Is a quote by which philosopher in his The Social Contract?

A) Jean-Jacque Rousseau
B) Voltaire
C) Karl Marx
D) Thomas Hobbes
E) John Locke

Question 5:
Argentina is named after what Element in the periodic table?

A) Gold
B) Silver
C) Lead
D) Carbon
E) Potassium

Question 6:
Whose national flag features a Cedar tree?

A) Greece
B) Jordan
C) Israel
D) Iraq
E) Lebanon

Question 7:
The death drive is a theory postulated by what 19th century founder of psychology?

A) Karl Jung
B) Sigmund Freud
C) William James
D) B. F Skinner
E) Ivan Pavlov

Question 8:
Constantinople and Byzantium are both previous names of what European city?

A) Athens
B) Rome
C) Florence
D) Istanbul
E) Split

Question 9:
'Bootlegging' in the 1920's America was a method of smuggling what?

A) Cigarettes
B) Tea
C) Lye
D) Alcohol
E) Cocaine

Question 10:
What do presidents Franklin D Roosevelt, John F Kennedy and William McKinley all have in common?

A) Died in office
B) Were impeached
C) Were assassinated
D) Were alcoholics
E) Resigned their office

Question 11:
The Bell Jar is a semi-autobiographical novel by which poet?

A) W.B Yeats
B) Emily Dickenson
C) Walt Whitman
D) Sylvia Plath
E) T. S. Eliot

Question 12:
The Stradivarius is the world's most expensive kind of what?

A) Watch
B) Violin
C) Boat
D) Piano
E) Car

Question 13:
A chemical change may add something to a substance, or subtract something from it, or it may both subtract and add, making a new substance with entirely different properties. Sulphur and carbon are two stable solids. The chemical union of the two forms a volatile liquid. A substance may be at one time a solid, at another a liquid, at another a gas, and yet not undergo any chemical change, because in each case the chemical composition is identical.

Which of the following statements cannot be reliably concluded from the above passage?

A) The chemical composition of a compound may influence its physical nature.
B) Substances can exist as solid, liquid or gas, without their chemical composition changing.
C) Chemicals can be combined to create a new substance with similar or very different properties.
D) Combining two substances in one state can lead to the production of a compound in a completely different state.
E) The transition from solid to liquid is not a chemical one.

Question 14:
An insect differs from a horse, for example, as much as a modern printing press differs from the press Franklin used. Both machines are made of iron, steel, wood, etc., and both print; but the plan of their structure differs throughout, and some parts are wanting in the simpler press, which are present and absolutely essential in the other. So with the two sorts of animals; they are built up originally out of protoplasm, or the original jelly-like germinal matter, which fills the cells composing their tissues, and nearly the same chemical elements occur in both, but the mode in which these are combined, the arrangement of their products: the muscular, nervous and skin tissues, differ in the two animals.

Which of the following statements can be reliably concluded from the above passage?

A) The printing press has adapted from the press Franklin used, due to the designers observing differences in nature.
B) Horses and insects differ as they are made up of completely different chemical elements.
C) The muscular, nervous and skin tissues are what define an organism.
D) Chemical elements make up protoplasm, which is the building block for all major organisms.
E) It is the manner in which chemicals are arranged that determine an organism as a final product.

Question 15:
What day comes two days after the day, which comes four days after the day, which comes immediately after the day, which comes two days before Monday?

A) Monday   B) Tuesday   C) Thursday   D) Saturday   E) Sunday

Question 16:
If John gives Michael £20, the ratio of their money is 2:1. If Michael gives John £5, the ratio of John's money to Michael's is 5:1. How much money do they have combined?

A) £180   B) £120   C) £90   D) £210   E) £150

Question 17:
From the primitive pine-torch to the paraffin candle, how wide an interval! Between them how vast a contrast! The means adopted by man to illuminate his home at night, stamp at once his position in the scale of civilisation. The fluid bitumen of the far East, blazing in rude vessels of baked earth; the Etruscan lamp, exquisite in form, yet ill adapted to its office; the whale, seal, or bear fat, filling the hut of the Esquimaux or Lap with odour rather than light; the huge wax candle on the glittering altar, the range of gas lamps in our streets, all have their stories to tell.

Which of the following statements best summarises the above passage?

A) Burning animal fat was the original way to produce fire.
B) The use of fire has spread to all corners of the Earth.
C) Using fire for light is what defines us as being human.
D) Each light source over the globe is able to tell its own tale.
E) The development and evolution of the use of fire helps to define mankind as a civilisation.

Question 18:
It was a little late to search for the philosophers' stone in 1669, yet it was in such a search that phosphorus was discovered. Wilhelm Homberg (1652-1715) described it in the following manner: "a man little known, of low birth, with a bizarre and mysterious nature in all he did, found this luminous matter while searching for something else."

What can be reliably concluded about the above passage?

A) Phosphorous was easy to identify as a result of its luminous nature.
B) Phosphorous was found as a result of this man's low social status.
C) Phosphorous was identified by accident, in the search for the philosophers' stone.
D) Wilhelm Homberg discovered phosphorous.
E) Phosphorous was discovered in the 18th century.

Question 19:
How many minutes past noon is it, if 3 times this many minutes before 3pm is 28 minutes later than this many minutes past noon?

A) 54   B) 32   C) 45   D) 38   E) 18

Question 20:

Everyone is familiar with the main facts of such a life-story as that of a moth or butterfly. The form of the adult insect is dominated by the wings—two pairs of scaly wings, carried respectively on the middle and hindmost of the three segments that make up the *thorax* or central region of the insect's body. Each of these three segments carries a pair of legs.

Which of the following statements can be concluded from the above statement?

A) The wings of the insects alternate patterns when the insect flies.
B) The wings that attach to the segments of the insect's body are the most prominent feature of the butterfly or moth.
C) Wings attach to each of the three segments of the thorax.
D) Moths and butterflies are very similar in that each segment of their thorax carries a pair of legs.
E) Scaly wings protect these creatures from predators.

Question 21:

In 2007 AD, Halley's Comet and Comet Encke were observed in the same calendar year. Halley's Comet is observed on average once every 73 years; Comet Encke is observed on average once every 104 years. Based on this, estimate the calendar year in which both Halley's Comet and Comet Encke are next observed in the same year.

A) 9559 AD   B) 2114 AD   C) 5643 AD   D) 3562 AD   E) 1757 AD

Question 22:

In a school there are 40 more girls than there are boys. The boys make up a percentage of 40% of the school. What is the number of students in the school?

A) 150   B) 200   C) 300   D) 500   E) 720

END OF SECTION

Section 2

Question 23:

Hydrogen Bicarbonate (HCO_3^-) acts as a buffer in the blood i.e. to keep the PH close to 7.

Which statement is true regarding bicarbonate?

A) It is alkaline.
B) It is an acidic molecule.
C) If the pH of the blood drops below 7, bicarbonate will release the H^+ ion to stabilise the pH.
D) It is only released when the pH drops below 7.
E) It is bound to protein in the blood.

Question 24:

The below statements are about breathing. Which of them are correct?

1. The diaphragm plays no part in breathing.
2. The intercostal muscles relax during exhalation to allow the ribcage to move inwards and downwards.
3. The total pressure inside the chest decreases relative to the pressure outside the body during inhaling to draw air inside the lungs.

A) 1 only
B) 2 only
C) 3 only

D) 2 and 3
E) 1 and 3
F) None

Question 25:

In pregnancy the foetus is supplied with blood from the mother via the umbilical cord. This cord is comprised of one vein and two arteries. The table below shows which vessel carries which type of blood in which direction.

	Vessel	Direction	Blood
1.	Vein	Mother to foetus	Oxygenated
2.	Artery	Foetus to Mother	Deoxygenated
3.	Artery	Foetus to Mother	Oxygenated
4.	Vein	Mother to Foetus	Deoxygenated

Which options are correct?

A) 1 only
B) 2 only

C) 3 only
D) 4 only

E) 1 and 2
F) 2 and 3

G) 4 and 1
H) 3 and 1

Question 26:

What is the function of the kidneys?

1. Ultrafiltration
2. Kill bacteria in the blood
3. Reabsorption
4. Release of waste

5. Store water
6. Produce hormones
7. Blood glucose regulation

A) 1 only
B) 2 only

C) 3 only
D) 4 only

E) 5 only
F) 6 and 7

G) 3 and 5
H) 1, 3 and 4

I) 4, 5 and 6

Question 27:
Mike and Vanessa are two healthy adults. They have two children. Their first child, Rory, was born with Haemophilia B, an X linked recessive disorder that causes problems with blood clotting. They have just had another baby, a girl and want to get her tested for the condition. What is the likelihood of the baby girl having the condition?

A) 0%   B) 25%   C) 50%   D) 75%   E) 34%

Question 28:
Bacteria invade the body and produce toxins that kill cells.

What are some of the first line defences the body has to prevent bacteria entering?
1. Mucus lining the airways
2. Heat produced by the body
3. Skin
4. Antibodies produced by the immune system
5. Toxins produced by the body
6. Hydrochloric acid in the stomach

A) 1 only   C) 3 only   E) 4, 5 and 6   G) 2 and 4
B) 2 only   D) 1, 3, 4 and 6   F) 1, 3 and 6

Question 29:
Which of the following is true with regards to osmosis?

A) It does not require a concentration gradient
B) It can apply to any substance, not just water
C) It is the movement of water across a partially permeable membrane
D) It is an active process
E) Transporters move water molecules across the membrane of cells

Question 30:
The carbon cycle is the cycle regarding the intake and release of carbon by organisms. Which of these statements are true?

A) Plants take carbon via photosynthesis and taking nutrients from the soil, which have come from decayed organisms.
B) Animals give off carbon via respiration, waste, eating and death.
C) The CO_2 in the air comes from burning of plant/animal products and respiration from living organisms only.
D) Trees do not store any carbon as they give it all off as carbon dioxide.

Question 31:
Enzymes are thought to work by two mechanisms – lock and key or the induced fit theory. The Lock and Key theory states that the active site of an enzyme is already perfectly shaped for the substrate, whereas the induced fit theory states that the enzyme's active site moulds itself around the substrate's shape. Which of these statements is true?

A) Enzymes are substrate specific.
B) The induced fit theory allows multiple, different types of substrates to be acted on by one enzyme.
C) The induced fit theory allows multiple, different types of enzymes to work on the same substrate.
D) The lock and key theory does not allow space for catatonic reactions (breaking the substrate up.

Questions 32-33 are based on the following information:
DNA is made up of the four nucleotide bases: adenine, cytosine, guanine and thymine. A triplet repeat or codon is a sequence of three nucleotides which code for an amino acid. While there are only 20 amino acids there are 64 different combinations of the four DNA nucleotide bases. This means that more than one combination of 3 DNA nucleotides sequences code for the same amino acid.

Question 32:
Which property of the DNA code is described above?

A) The code is unambiguous.
B) The code is universal.
C) The code is non-overlapping.
D) The code is degenerate.
E) The code is preserved.
F) The code has no punctuation.

Question 33:
Which type of mutation does the described property protect against the most?
A) An insertion - where a single nucleotide is inserted.
B) A point mutation - where a single nucleotide is replaced for another.
C) A deletion - where a single nucleotide is deleted.
D) A repeat expansion - where a repeated trinucleotide sequence is added.
E) A duplication - where a piece of DNA is abnormally copied.

Question 34:
Which of the following processes involve active transport?

1. Reabsorption of glucose in the kidney.
2. Movement of carbon dioxide into the alveoli in the lungs.
3. Movement of chemicals in a neural synapse.

A) 1 only
B) 2 only
C) 3 only
D) 1 and 2
E) 1 and 3
F) 2 and 3
G) 1, 2 and 3

Question 35:
Which of the following statements is correct about enzymes?

A) All enzymes are made up of amino acids only.
B) Enzymes can sometimes slow the rate of reactions.
C) Enzymes have no impact on reaction temperatures.
D) Enzymes are heat sensitive but resistant to changes in pH.
E) Enzymes are unspecific in their substrate use.
F) None of the above.

Question 36:
Which of the following statements about the Krebs cycle are correct?

1. Three molecules of reduced NAD and one molecule of reduced FAD are produced each turn
2. Citric acid is regenerated to be used in the next cycle
3. ATP can be produced by substrate-level phosphorylation

A) 1
B) 2
C) 3
D) 1 and 2
E) 1 and 3
F) 1, 2 and 3

Question 37:

Which of the following statements about the light-dependent reaction are correct?

1. Cyclic phosphorylation uses photosystems I and II
2. Non-cyclic phosphorylation produces ATP, NADPH and oxygen
3. Water is required for both cyclic and non-cyclic photophosphorylation

A) 1
B) 2
C) 3
D) 1 and 2
E) 1 and 3
F) 1, 2 and 3

Question 38:

Which of the following statements about the Calvin cycle are correct?

1. RUBISCO is a co-enzyme
2. It requires 6 turns of he Calvin cycle to make 1 glucose molecules
3. Fatty acids can be synthesised from glycerate-3-phosphate

A) 1
B) 2
C) 2 and 3
D) 1 and 3
E) 1, 2 and 3
F) None of them

Question 39:

Which of the following statements about action potentials are correct?

1. Depolarisation is driven by an influx of sodium ions
2. Hyperpolarisation makes action potentials unidirectional
3. The speed of an action potential depends on the temperature and the diameter of the axon

A) 1
B) 2
C) 3
D) 1 and 2
E) 1 and 3
F) 1, 2 and 3

Question 40:

A patient has been diagnosed with type 1 diabetes. Which statements about hormonal control of glucose are correct?

1. Insulin injections need to be closely monitored to prevent hypoglycaemia
2. Adrenaline increases the storage of glucose as glycogen
3. Glucagon is released from α-cells of the pancreas in response to a fall in blood glucose

END OF SECTION

Section 3

Question 41:

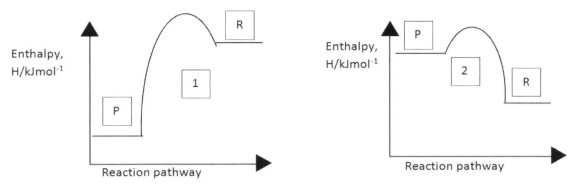

The two graphs shown above are Enthalpy profile diagrams. Which best describes an endothermic reaction?

	Graph	ΔH	Heat energy	Stability of reactants
A)	1	Negative	Absorbed from surroundings	P is more stable than R
B)	2	Negative	Released to surroundings	R is more stable than P
C)	1	Positive	Absorbed from surroundings	P is more stable than R
D)	2	Positive	Absorbed from surroundings	R is more stable than P

Question 42:

Pyrite, also known as Fool's Gold, is an ore of Iron containing sulphur in the form of iron (II) disulphide, FeS_2. By mass 75% of this ore is FeS_2.

Calculate the maximum mass of iron that can be extracted from 480kg of ore.
[A_r: Fe = 55; S = 32]

A) 167.7kg   B) 200kg   C) 360.5kg   D) 118kg   E) 120.2kg

Question 43:

$X_{(s)} + FeSO_{4(aq)} \rightarrow XSO_{4(aq)} + Fe_{(s)}$

Which metal can be correctly be substituted in X's place?

A) Tin (Sn)   C) Lead (Pb)   E) Copper (Cu)
B) Zinc (Zn)   D) Silver (Ag)

Question 44:

Which of the following statements about catalysts are true?

1. Catalysts reduce the energy required for a reaction to take place.
2. Catalysts are used up in reactions.
3. Catalysed reactions are almost always exothermic.

A. 1 only   B. 2 only   C. 1 and 2   D. 2 and 3   E. 1, 2 and 3

Question 45:
The element shown below is Germanium. It has an ionic charge of 4+. How many electrons does one atom of Germanium have?

| 73 |
| Ge |
| 32 |

A) 32   B) 73   C) 36   D) 41   E) 4

Question 46:
For the following reaction, which of the statements is true?
$CH_{4(g)} + 2O_{2(g)} \rightarrow 2H_2O_{(aq)} + CO_{2(g)}$

A) This is an example of complete combustion.
B) By increasing the concentration of CO_2 you can increase the rate of combustion
C) The reaction is anaerobic
D) Combustion of a gas always produces a liquid like water
E) If you remove some of the oxygen you get more product.

Question 47:
Which of the following statements is true?
1. Ethane and ethene can both dissolve in organic solvents.
2. Ethane and ethene can both be hydrogenated in the presence of Nickel.
3. Breaking C=C requires double the energy needed to break C-C.

A. 1 only   C. 3 only   E. 2 and 3 only   G. 1, 2 and 3
B. 2 only   D. 1 and 2 only   F. 1 and 3 only

Question 48:
Diamond, Graphite, Methane and Ammonia all exhibit covalent bonding. Which row adequately describes the properties associated with each?

	Compound	Melting Point	Able to conduct electricity	Soluble in water
1.	Diamond	High	Yes	No
2.	Graphite	High	Yes	No
3.	$CH_{4(g)}$	Low	No	No
4.	$NH_{3(g)}$	Low	No	Yes

A. 1 and 2 only   D. 1 and 4 only   G. 1,2 and 4
B. 2 and 3 only   E. 1, 2 and 3   H. 1, 2, 3 and 4
C. 1 and 3 only   F. 2, 3 and 4

Question 49:

What is the name of the molecule below?

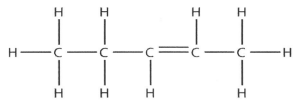

A. But-1-ene
B. But-2-ene

C. Pent-3-ene
D. Pent-1-ene

E. Pent-2-ene
F. Pentane

G. Pentanoic acid

Question 50:

Which of the following statements is correct regarding Group 1 elements? [Excluding Hydrogen]

A. The oxidation number of Group 1 elements usually decreases in most reactions.
B. Reactivity decreases as you progress down Group 1.
C. Group 1 elements do not react with water.
D. All Group 1 elements react spontaneously with oxygen.
E. All of the above.
F. None of the above.

Question 51:

Which of the following statements about electrolysis are correct?

1. The cathode attracts negatively charged ions.
2. Atoms are reduced at the anode.
3. Electrolysis can be used to separate mixtures.

A. Only 1
B. Only 2
C. Only 3

D. 1 and 2
E. 2 and 3
F. 1 and 3

G. 1, 2 and 3
H. None of the above.

Question 52:

Which of the following is **NOT** an isomer of pentane?

A. $CH_3CH_2CH_2CH_2CH_3$
B. $CH_3C(CH_3)CH_3CH_3$

C. $CH_3(CH_2)_3CH_3$
D. $CH_3C(CH_3)_2CH_3$

END OF SECTION

Section 4

Question 53:

Which of the statements regarding this series circuit is true?

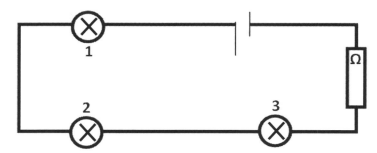

A) Current is different at different points in the circuit.
B) Potential difference is shared between the three lightbulbs.
C) Resistance is constant throughout the circuit.
D) The current is higher in bulb 1 than in bulbs 2 and 3.

Question 54:

Bill wants to lay down laminate flooring in his living room, which has an in-built circular fish tank that he will have to lay the flooring around. He has decided to buy planks that he can cut to fit the dimensions of his room. He must, however, buy whole planks and cut them down himself. The room's dimensions are given below, as are those of one plank.

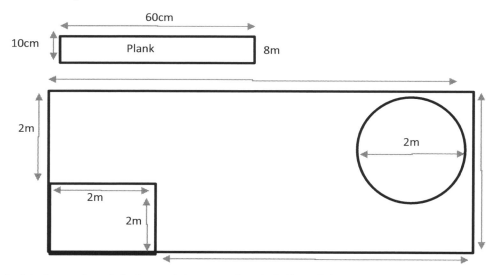

Calculate the number of planks needed to cover the whole floor. Take $\pi = 3$.

  A) 30   B) 417   C) 600   D) 589   E) 43

Question 55:

Solve $y = x^2 - 3x + 4$ and $y - x = 1$ as (x,y).

A) (-1, 2) and (3,4)   C) (7,-2) and (6,5)   E) (1,-1) and (-7,-1)
B) (1,2) and (3,4)   D) (2,-3) and (4,-1)

Question 56:
A ball of mass 5kg is at rest at the top of a 5m slope. Calculate the velocity of the ball as it travels down the slope. Take $g = 10kgm^{-1}$ and assume there is no resistance.

A) 10   B) 45   C) 100   D) 5   E) 6

Question 57:
Which of the following statements is true regarding Red Shift?

A) The further a distant galaxy or celestial object is, the further down the red end of the light spectrum it's light will be.
B) The closer a galaxy gets, the longer it's wavelengths get, thus moving down the red end of the spectrum.
C) Red shift means that we never see the real light from distant galaxies.
D) We can never tell how far away galaxies are using red shift.

Question 58:
Which is true regarding X-rays?

A) X-rays do not pass through denser materials like bone and that's why they show up as white on the X-ray film.
B) X-rays pass through bone but not skin and soft tissue, and that's why bones show up white on the X-ray film.
C) X-rays don't ionise cells and thus are safe.
D) Gamma rays are safer than X-rays.

Question 59:
Rearrange $\frac{(16x+11)}{(4x+5)} = 4y^2 + 2$ to make x the subject

A) $x = \frac{20y^2-1}{[16-4\,(4y^2+2)]}$ C) $= \frac{6y^2-1}{[16-4\,(4y^2+2)]}$ E) $= \frac{7y^2-1}{[6-14\,(6+7)]}$

B) $= \frac{20y^2-8}{[16-6\,(4y^2+2)]}$ D) $= \frac{21y^2-1}{[16-4\,(2y^2+2)]}$

Question 60:
If $(3p + 5)^2 = 24p + 49$, calculate p.

A) -5 or -9   B) -3 or -6   C) -4 or 6   D) -6 or 4   E) 4 or -2

END OF PAPER

ANSWERS

ANSWER KEY

PAPER E							
Section 1		**Section 2**		**Section 3**		**Section 4**	
1	B	23	F	41	E	53	D
2	C	24	D	42	F	54	A
3	A	25	A	43	F	55	C
4	C	26	C	44	B	56	D
5	B	27	E	45	E	57	B
6	A	28	F	46	B	58	C
7	A	29	E	47	D	59	E
8	E	30	B	48	D	60	B
9	C	31	B	49	D		
10	A	32	F	50	D		
11	A	33	E	51	E		
12	B	34	B	52	E		
13	C	35	A				
14	B	36	I				
15	C	37	C				
16	E	38	B				
17	D	39	D				
18	A	40	A				
19	D						
20	E						
21	D						
22	B+E						

PAPER F							
Section 1		**Section 2**		**Section 3**		**Section 4**	
1	A	23	G	41	A	53	F
2	B	24	E	42	C	54	D
3	D	25	C	43	A	55	A
4	C	26	C	44	C	56	B
5	D	27	C	45	H	57	B
6	A	28	D	46	B	58	C
7	D	29	E	47	B	59	A
8	B	30	B	48	G	60	B
9	A	31	C	49	A		
10	E	32	D	50	B		
11	E	33	C	51	E		
12	A	34	C	52	B		
13	D	35	A				
14	A	36	B				
15	C	37	C				
16	B	38	B				
17	C	39	F				
18	D	40	E				
19	D						
20	D						
21	B						
22	E						

PAPER G							
Section 1		**Section 2**		**Section 3**		**Section 4**	
1	B	23	B	41	H	53	D
2	B	24	D	42	B	54	B
3	A	25	E	43	A	55	B
4	C	26	A	44	F	56	B
5	C	27	D	45	E	57	B
6	B	28	A	46	A	58	E
7	C	29	B	47	C	59	B
8	B	30	D	48	D	60	C
9	C	31	D	49	A		
10	A	32	A	50	A		
11	D	33	A	51	B		
12	C	34	A	52	B		
13	C	35	C				
14	E	36	A				
15	E	37	F				
16	E	38	F				
17	C	39	E				
18	B	40	D				
19	A						
20	D						
21	D						
22	B						

PAPER H							
Section 1		**Section 2**		**Section 3**		**Section 4**	
1	D	23	A	41	C	53	B
2	D	24	D	42	A	54	B
3	C	25	E	43	B	55	B
4	A	26	H	44	A	56	A
5	B	27	A	45	A	57	A
6	E	28	F	46	A	58	A
7	B	29	C	47	A	59	A
8	D	30	B	48	F	60	D
9	D	31	A	49	E		
10	A	32	D	50	D		
11	D	33	B	51	H		
12	B	34	A	52	B		
13	A	35	F				
14	E	36	E				
15	D	37	B				
16	E	38	C				
17	E	39	F				
18	C	40	E				
19	D						
20	B						
21	D						
22	A						

Mock Paper E Answers

Question 1: B
Sao Paolo, Rio De Janeiro and Brasilia are all important Brazilian cities. Brasilia was made the Administrative Capital of Brazil. It was planned and built in the 1950s to replace Rio De Janeiro.

Question 2: C
Although all are notable German thinkers, Marx and Engels wrote the Communist Manifesto.

Question 3: A
While all these islands had early Greek settlements on them, Crete was home to the Minoan civilisation, one of the oldest civilisations on Earth, with its own distinctive culture and art style.

Question 4: C
Named after the Medieval friar William of Occam, and still an important principle today in science and philosophy, Occam's Razor states that 'All things being equal, given two possible explanations the simplest is preferred.' Example: If a glass of water is knocked over when I am not home I could deduce it was either A) My cat, or B) Ghosts. The best explanation is that my cat did it, as it does not require me to explain what ghosts are, why I think they exist, how they can knock things overly with their ghostly hands etc.

Question 5: B
Wordsworth, Keats and Byron were all Romantic poets, John Donne and Shakespeare belong to the Elizabethan period. Wordworth is sometimes considered one of the founders of Romanticism, a great admirer of nature. I wandered lonely as a cloud

> *I wandered lonely as a cloud*
> *That floats on high o'er vales and hills,*
> *When all at once I saw a crowd,-*
> *A host, of golden daffodils;*
> *Beside the lake, beneath the trees,*
> *Fluttering and dancing in the breeze.*

Question 6: A
Henry Kissinger was awarded the Nobel peace prize in 1973, causing several committee members to resign in protest.

Question 7: A
The British Labour party was formed in 1900 amid growing concern for labour rights worldwide. The Whig and Conservative party are far older. The Green party has its origins in the People's Party, formed in 1972, and the Liberal Democrats were formed in the 1980's by a merger between the SDP and the Liberal Party.

Question 8: E
The Motherboard is the central component of a computer. It has some alternative names including Mainboard, Logicboard and Systemboard. Megatron is the nemesis of Optimus Prime in the original Transformers cartoon series.

Question 9: C
Nelson was a very famous admiral by the time of his death at the battle of Trafalgar. Waterloo was a decisive land battle during the Napoleonic wars.

Question 10: A
Having been shown a prototype of an Apple computer in 1976 Steve Jobs founded Apple Computers. Steve Jobs also founded Pixar in 1986, acquiring the graphics division of Lucasfilm Ltd and renaming it.

Question 11: A
The famous Cogito, I think therefore I am, was written by Rene Descartes in his Meditations, in which he tried to establish what it was possible to know for certain.

Question 12: B
Bits of the Sistine Chapel were painted by multiple painters including Botticelli, Perugino and Ghirlandaio. The ceiling itself though, and the Creation of Adam, was painted by Michelangelo.

Question 13: C
Tom arrives at 1620, and leaves 45 mins after Jane leaves. Therefore he also leaves 45 mins after Hannah leaves, since Jane and Hannah leave together. Since his journey is 10 mins faster than Hannah's, he arrives only 35 minutes after Hannah arrives (which happens to be 1620). Therefore Hannah arrives 35 minutes earlier than this, at 1545. Since she left at 1430, her journey took 75 minutes. Jane's journey took 40% longer (1.4 x 75 = 105 minutes). Therefore leaving at the same time as Hannah, 1430, Jane arrived 105 minutes later at 1615.

Question 14: B
This is a simultaneous equations question. Let **x** be the number of standard tickets sold, and **y** be the number of premium tickets sold.
Therefore: $x + y = 600$; $10x + 16y = 6{,}600$
$x = 600 - y$ » substitute: $10(600 - y) + 16y = 6600$
$6y = 600$
$y = 100$, therefore 100 premium tickets were sold.

Question 15: C
Between 20th January and 23rd May, there are 123 days. In 123 days, the moon makes $123/28 = 4.39$ orbits. This is equal to $4.39 \times 360° = 1580°$

Question 16: E
You are looking for a strong opposition to the proposition that students at drama academies are not taught well academically. The strongest opposition would be evidence that such students perform academically well in some objective measure. Evidence of significantly above average GCSE results provides this.

Question 17: D
You should definitely draw this one out on paper. Trace out the paths and you find that both people have a net displacement of 11km to the North. Therefore since Anil is only net 2km East, and Suresh is 17km East of the starting point, there is a 15km separation between them

Question 18: A
Walking at 4mph, 3 miles takes ¾ hour = 45 mins. Adding the 5 minute stop, Chris will arrive at 1820, since he set off at 1730. At 24mph, 6 miles takes ¼ hour, 15 mins. Therefore setting off at 1810, Sarah will arrive at Laura's at 1825. Therefore Chris arrives 5 minutes earlier than Sarah.

Question 19: D
The passage tells us that illegal downloads are causing harm to the music industry. Whilst it gives an example, this does not mean the stated example is the principal issue. The conclusion that best fits the passage as a whole is to say illegal downloading is more harmful than many people think, given their willingness to undertake it.

Question 20: E

First, calculate the amount of water needed for each type of fire. Use algebra:

Use x as the amount of water used to extinguish a house fire. 40,000L = 2x , so x = 20,000L. Then, take y as the amount of water needed to extinguish a garden fire, so 70,000L = 2x + 3y. 30,000L = 3y, y= 10,000L.

Knowing this, A is correct, B is correct, C is correct and D is correct. Only E is false.

Three house and ten garden fires require 160,000 litres to extinguish, not 140,000.

Question 21: D

The passage only talks about people's opinions on the scheme, and not about any action which could potentially be taken. Therefore the best summary is to say that more people oppose the scheme than support it.

Question 22: B + E

The question asks for two responses, therefore you must mark two and get them both correct for one mark. The suggestion is made that reducing wild fishing will improve fish populations. This assertion carries two major assumptions – that the fishing originally caused the decline, and that the decline is reversible, and can therefore recover if the threat is removed. Select these two responses for a mark.

Question 23: F

None of the above, they are all true facts about digestion.

Question 24: D

Blood flow to the kidneys is constant - not exercise dependent. Overall cardiac output increases since heart rate and stroke volume increase (because there is greater oxygen demand from exercising muscle). There is more blood flow to the muscles to fuel them and to the skin to help lose excess heat. Blood flow to the gut decreases to increase availability to muscles. Blood flow to vital organs such as the kidney and brain remains constant.

Question 25: A

Since A-T and C-G are the DNA base pairings, 29.6% Adenine implies 29.6% Thymine as well. Therefore the remaining 100 – 59.2 = 40.8% is shared between Guanine and Cytosine equally, so there is 20.4% cytosine.

Question 26: C

Since CO binds to the oxygen binding site of haemoglobin, it reduces oxygen binding and therefore oxygen carrying capacity of blood. Hence, the blood becomes less oxygenated. Since more blood needs to flow to deliver the same amount of oxygen, this must be accomplished by an increased in heart rate. Haemoglobin does not become heavier as the CO binds **instead** of oxygen rather than in **addition** to. Carbon Dioxide is carried in plasma so is unaffected by carbon monoxide poisoning which affects haemoglobin.

Question 27: E

The most effective method in minimising side effects would be to only target bacteria. Only bacteria have a flagellum.

Question 28: F

Structure A is the right semi-lunar valve, the pulmonary valve. It opens in systole to allow flow of blood from the right ventricle into the pulmonary artery and to the lungs. It closes in diastole to ensure the right ventricle fills only from the right atrium, maintaining a one-way flow of blood. Therefore F is true, it opens when the right atrium is emptying. None of the other statements are true.

Question 29: E

E is the correct sequence. Remember sensory neurone take sensory information to the brain, and motor neurones take information away.

Question 30: B

Intra-thoracic volume must decrease during expiration. Thus, the intercostal muscles relax causing the ribs must move down and in. The diaphragm moves up as well.

Question 31: B

If lipase is not working, fat from the diet will not be broken down, and will build up in the stool. Lactase, for instance, is responsible for breaking down lactose, and its malfunctioning causes lactose-intolerance.

Question 32: F

Oxygenated blood flows from the lungs to the heart via the pulmonary vein. The pulmonary artery carries deoxygenated blood from the heart to the lungs. Animals like fish have single circulatory systems. Deoxygenated blood is found in the superior vena cava, returning to the heart from the body. Veins in the arms and hands frequently don't have valves.

Question 33: E

Enzymatic digestion takes place throughout the GI tract, including in the mouth (e.g. amylase), stomach (e.g. pepsin), and small intestine (e.g. trypsin). The large intestine is primarily responsible for water absorption, whilst the rectum acts as a temporary store for faecal matter (i.e. digestion has finished by the rectum).

Question 34: B

This is an example of the monosynaptic stretch reflex; these reflexes are performed at the spinal level and therefore don't involve the brain.

Question 35: A

Statement 2 describes diffusion, as CO_2 is moving with the concentration gradient. Statement 3 describes active transport, as amino acids are moving against the concentration gradient.

Question 36: I

3 is the correct equation for animals, and 4 is correct for plants.

Question 37: C

The mitochondria are only the site for aerobic respiration, as anaerobic respiration occurs in the cytoplasm. Aerobic respiration produces more ATP per substrate than anaerobic respiration, and therefore is also more efficient. The chemical equation for glucose being respired aerobically is: $C_6H_{12}O_6 + 6O_2 \rightarrow 6CO_2 + 6H_2O$. Thus, the molar ratio is 1:6 (i.e. each mole glucose produces 6 moles of CO_2).

Question 38: B

The nucleus contains the DNA and chromosomes of the cell. The cytoplasm contains enzymes, salts and amino acids in addition to water. The plasma membrane is a bilayer. Lastly, the cell wall is indeed responsible for protecting vs. increased osmotic pressures.

Question 39: D

When a medium is hypertonic relative to the cell cytoplasm, it is more concentrated than the cytoplasm, and when it is hypotonic, it is less concentrated. So, when a medium is hypotonic relative to the cell cytoplasm, the cell will gain water through osmosis. When the medium is isotonic, there will be no net movement of water across the cell membrane. Lastly, when the medium is hypertonic relative to the cell cytoplasm, the cell will lose water by osmosis.

Question 40: A

Stem cells have the ability to differentiate and produce other kinds of cells. However, they also have the ability to generate cells of their own kind and stem cells are able to maintain their undifferentiated state. The two types of stem cells are embryonic stem cells and adult stem cells. The adult stem cells are present in both children and adults.

Question 41: E

Recall that reduction is the gain of electrons whilst oxidation is a loss. Also remember that oxidation the gain of oxygen, while reduction is loss. Only Iodine is gaining electrons and so shows reduction.

Question 42: F

To balance the equation, start working from what you're given – the oxygen. Since you know there are 15 oxygen atoms on the right, there must be the same on the left. Therefore **w** = 5. You also know that there are 30 Hydrogen atoms on the right hand side, and so you can work out x. 30-5 leaves 25 atoms unaccounted for, so x=25.

Question 43: F

The information given can only be used to work out the empirical formula. You would need to know the molar mass in order to calculate the chemical formula.

Question 44: B

The trick in this question is to conserve your units to prevent silly mistakes from creeping in. $200\ cm^{-3} = 0.2\ dm^{-3}$

$Number\ of\ moles\ =\ concentration\ x\ volume$ so: $0.2\ x\ 1.8\ =\ 0.36\ mol$

Question 45: E

Group 6 elements are non-metals whilst group 3 elements are metals. Thus, the group 3 element must lose electrons when it reacts with the group 6 element. The donation of electrons from its outer shell will decrease atomic size.

Question 46: B

Reactivity of both group 1 and 2 increases as you go down the groups because the valence electrons that react are further away from the positively charged nucleus (which means the electrostatic attraction between them is weaker). Group 1 metals are usually more reactive because they only need to donate one electron, whilst group 2 metals must donate two electrons.

Question 47: D

This is a straightforward question that tests basic understanding of kinetics. Catalysts help overcome energy barriers by reducing the activation energy necessary for a reaction.

Question 48: D

H^1 contains 1 proton and no neutrons. Isotopes have the same numbers of protons, but different numbers of neutrons. Thus, H^3 contains two more neutrons than H^1.

Question 49: D

These statements all come from the Kinetic Theory of Gases, an idealised model of gases that allows for the derivation of the ideal gas law. The angle at which gas molecules move is not related to temperature; movement is random. Gas molecules lose no energy when they collide with each other, collisions are assumed elastic. The average kinetic energy of gas molecules is the same for all gases at the same temperature as they are assumed to be point masses. Momentum = mass x velocity. Therefore, the momentum of gas molecules increases with pressure as a greater force is exerted on each molecule.

Question 50: D

Oxidation is the loss of electrons and reduction is the gain of electrons (therefore increasing electron density). Halogens tend to act as electron recipients in reactions and are therefore good oxidising agents.

Question 51: E

An exothermic reaction is defined as a chemical reaction that releases energy. Thus, aerobic respiration producing life energy, the burning of magnesium, and the reacting of acids/bases are almost always exothermic processes. Similarly, the combustion of most things (including hydrogen) is exothermic. Evaporation of water is a physical process in which no chemical reaction is taking place.

Question 52: E

$2 C_3H_6 + 9 O_2 \rightarrow 6 H_2O + 6 CO_2$

Assign the oxidation numbers for each element:

For C_3H_6: $C = -2$; $H = +1$

For O_2: $O = 0$

For H_2O: $H = +1$; $O = -2$

For CO_2: $C = +4$; $O = -2$

Look for the changes in the oxidation numbers:

H remained at $+1$

C changed from -2 to $+4$. Thus, it was oxidized

O changed from 0 to -2. Thus, it was reduced.

Question 53: D

Firstly, convert Litres $\rightarrow$ m^3: 950 Litres = 0.95 m^3

Buoyancy Force = Volume x Density x g.

= 0.95 x 1000 x 10 = 9,500 N

Weight of the boat = mg= 600 x 10 = 6,000 N

Since buoyancy force > Weight, the boat will float.

The difference between Buoyancy Force + weight = 9500 – 6000 = 3,500N

Hence adding mass of 350kg (=3,500N as g is 10) will balance both forces.

Adding further mass will cause the boat to sink. Hence, the answer is 355kg (350kg won't cause sinking – merely balance the force).

Question 54: A

Remember that you can separate the vertical and horizontal components of both bullets. Both bullets actually have zero vertical velocity at t=0. Thus, only gravity affects them- and it does so equally. Therefore, rather counter-intuitively, they hit the floor at the same time.

Question 55: C

You don't need to know the mass of the fish for this one, since there is no acceleration or deceleration taking place. The resistive forces are equivalent to the force of thrust of the fish. Recall that work done = force x distance. Travelling at $2ms^{-1}$, the fish travels 60 seconds x 60 minutes x 2 ms^{-1} = 7200 m in one hour. Therefore the work done against resistive forces is f x d = 2N x 7200 = <u>14,400J</u>

Question 56: D

A Moment of force = Force x Perpendicular distance to pivot

If the lifting arm is a uniform 5m long, the weight exerts $2000 \ x \ 10 \ x \ 5 \ = \ 100,000 \ Nm$ of torque. In addition, there is a $250 \ x \ 10 \ x \ 2.5 \ = \ 6,250 \ Nm$ contribution from the weight of the beam ($\frac{5}{7}$ the mass, acting through the centre of mass of the beam).

On the other side, the remaining $\frac{2}{7}$ of the beam makes a $100 \ x \ 10 \ x \ 1 \ = \ 1,000 \ Nm$ contribution.

Therefore, the counterbalance must make a $(100,000 \ + \ 6,250) - 1,000 \ = \ 105,250 \ Nm$ contribution. As the counterbalance arm is 2 m long, this requires a weight of $\frac{105,250}{2} \ = \ 52,625 \ N$ weight, or a mass of 5,263 kg.

The crane's height is a distracter and not needed for this question

Question 57: B

Work out the total energy transferred - 20 x 50W =1,000W of overall power by the 20 strings of lights when on. As W = Js^{-1}, can use the time the lights are on to find the energy used over this time period. 8pm – 6am is 10 hours, so in seconds is 10x60x60 = 36,000s. When multiplying this by the power of all sets of lights, gives the energy used as:

1000 W x 36,000 s = 36,000,000 J of energy, or 36,000kJ. Multiply this by 20 to account for the lights being on for 20 days = gives 720,000 kJ

As 100 kJ of energy costs 2p, need to do 720,000/100 = 7,200. Multiply this by 2p = 14,400p. Convert to pounds by dividing by 100 = **£144.**

Question 58: C
The formula for the sum of internal angles in a regular polygon is given by: $180(n-2)$, where n is the number of sides of the polygon.
Thus: $180(n-2) = 150 \, x \, n$
$180n - 360 = 150n$
$3n = 36$
$n = 12$
Each side is 15cm so the perimeter is 12 x 15cm = 180cm.

Question 59: E
For Resistors in parallel, $\frac{1}{R_T} = \frac{R_1 \, x \, R_2 \ldots}{R_1 + R_2 \ldots}$

For the first segment: $\frac{1}{R} = \frac{1}{Z} + \frac{1}{Z} = \frac{2}{Z}$

For the second segment: $\frac{1}{R} = \frac{1}{Z} + \frac{1}{Z} + \frac{1}{Z} = \frac{3}{Z}$

For the third segment: $R = Z$

Thus the total resistance is: $Z + \frac{Z}{2} + \frac{Z}{3} = 22.$

$\frac{6Z + 3Z + 2Z}{6} = 22$

$11Z = 22 \, x \, 6$

$Z = \frac{132}{11} = 12 M\Omega$

Question 60: B
The volume of candle burned in 0.5 hour $= 0.5 \, x \, (\pi \, x \, 2^2) = 6cm^{-3}$

$6cm^{-3} = 6 \, x \, 10^{-3} \, m^3$

Since $Density = \frac{mass}{volume}$, in this case $900 \, kgm^{-3} = \frac{mass}{6 \, x \, 10^{-3} \, m^3}$

Thus, Mass burned $= 900 \, x \, 6 \, x \, 10^{-3} = 5400 \, x \, 10^{-3} kg = 5.4 \, g$

The Mr of $C_{24}H_{52} = 12 \, x \, 24 + 52 \, x \, 1 = 340.$

Thus the number of moles burned $= \frac{5.4}{340} = 0.016 \, moles.$

Total Energy transferred $= 0.016 \, x \, 11,000$

$= 16 \, x \, 10^{-3} \, x \, 11 \, x \, 10^3 = 11 \, x \, 16$

$= 176 \, kJ = 175,000 \, J$

END OF PAPER

Mock Paper F Answers

Question 1: A
Oumuamua is Hawaiian for 'scout'. Io is one of Jupiter's moons, Hammurabi was an ancient king, Akua is a Hawaiian word meaning God, and Maui is one of Hawaii's main islands.

Question 2: B
Leda was seduced by Zeus as a swan. Zeus changed into many things to seduce his lovers, including a cloud. He changed into a bull to seduce another lover, Europa.

Question 3: D
Hampton Court palace was home to Cardinal Wolsey, until Henry VIII saw it and claimed it for himself, the cardinal fearing execution gave his home up. It has been used by the royal family ever since.

Question 4: C
It measures windspeed. Anemo comes from the Greek anemos, meaning wind.

Question 5: D
The Taiping rebellion was a movement in China against the ruling Qing dynasty during the mid-19th century.

Question 6: A
Charles Darwin used the Galapagos islands to study evolution directly.

Question 7: D

Although their methods were slightly different, both men invented calculus synonymously leading to and fierce international dispute over who had been first.

Question 8: B
The Peterloo massacre occurred in Manchester when a rally for parliamentary representation was charged government cavalry. The rally had occurred in the wake of a difficult period in British history with widespread famine and unemployment.

Question 9: A
Although the aforementioned countries are not all in the Euro they are all EU members apart from Switzerland which has chosen to remain independent.

Question 10: E
The prophet Zoroaster who lived preached in Iran, taught of one God, a heaven, a hell, and gave a code of rules. While its precise foundation date is unknown, Zoroastrianism is old enough to have influenced all the Judaeo-Christian religions.

Question 11: E
India has 22 officially recognised languages, with Hindi being the most widely spoken. Pashto is a language spoken largely in Afghanistan.

Question 12: A
John F Kennedy was in office when the Cuban missile crisis occurred in 1962. His talks with Khrushchev averted a potential catastrophe.

Question 13: D

C is completely irrelevant, so is not a flaw. B is not a flaw because when assessing an argument, anything that is stated (i.e. not concluded from other reasons in the passage) is accepted as true. We do not require evidence or sources for any statistics presented. A and E are both claiming that something is immoral, which is thus expressing an opinion on the part of the arguer. This is not a flaw, the arguer is at liberty to claim something is immoral, and to claim that the government is morally obliged to act, and that it has not done so. Also, E claims that *arguably* this is the most outrageous flaw of the government, clearly expressing an opinion, which is thus not required to be supported. However, D identifies a valid flaw. The argument rests on us accepting that if there were less uninsured drivers, there would be less crashes. This is not necessarily correct, so D is a flaw in the passage.

Question 14: A

The sentence 'Thus, the situation in Brazil is not applicable to the UK, and legalising gun ownership in the UK would be a bad move' gives the main conclusion of the argument and this is summarised in A.B is partially supported by the passage, but the main conclusion concerns the situation in the UK and the passage states that there is little black market in the UK. C is incorrect as the passage only talks about gun ownership, not violent crime more generally. D is not fully supported by the passage, which states only that legalising guns would result in it being *easier* for criminals to acquire guns, not that there would be a large increase in their number. E is not the main conclusion as it focuses on an aspect of the evidence from Brazil, rather than the main conclusion which focuses on gun legislation in the UK.

Question 15: C

For each of the walls where there is no door, the wall is 6 tiles high and 5 tiles wide, which is 30 tiles. The wall where the door is requires a row of 2 tiles above the door, then there is a width of wall of 120cm which requires completely tiling, which is 6 tiles high and 3 tiles wide, hence this wall requires a total of 20 tiles. Hence a total of 110 tiles are required for the walls. The floor is 2 metres by 2 metres, so 5 tiles by 5 tiles, hence 25 tiles are required for the floor. Hence the answer is 135.

Question 16: B

Let the number of minutes the journey takes be t. Therefore, ABC charge $400+15t$ pence for the journey. We can calculate that XYZ taxis charge $400+(30\times6)$ pence, $= 580$ pence. Therefore, for both journeys to cost the same, $580=400+15t$. $180=15t$, therefore $t=12$. Therefore the 6 mile journey needs to take 12 minutes. 6 miles in 12 minutes is 30 miles per hour, so the answer is B.

Question 17: C

A, B, D and E are all directly stated in the passage, so can all be reliably concluded. Perhaps the trickiest of these to see is answer D, which is true because the passage says "*due to*" the advent of more accurate technology, thus clearly identifying that this had *caused* the switch to the situation of most watches being made by machine. C, however, is *not* necessarily true. The passage states that most *watches* are produced by machines, but only states that *some* watchmakers now only perform repairs. This does not necessarily mean that most watchmakers do not produce watches. It could be that only a handful are required in the entirety of the watch industry for repairs, and that the numbers still producing watches exceeds those in the repair business. Thus, C cannot be reliably concluded from the passage.

Question 18: D

Usually bread rolls cost 30p for a pack, but if the cost per bread roll is reduced by 1p then they will cost 24p. Hence we need to find z, where $24(z+1)=30z$, where z is the original number of packs that could have been afforded. $24z+24=30z$, hence $24=6z$, so $z=4$. Hence he was originally supposed to be buying 4 packets of bread rolls, which is 6 x 4 = 24 rolls.

Question 19: D

We can first work out the rate of girls' absenteeism. First we need to work out how many of the pupils at Heather Park Academy and Holland Wood Comprehensive are girls. Let g be the number of girls in Heather Park Academy. Then 0.06(g)+0.05(1000-g)=(1000)(0.056). Then 0.06g-0.05g=56-50. Then 0.01g=6, so g = 600. Hence 600 pupils at Heather Park Academy are girls. The proportions at Holland Wood Comprehensive are the same but there are half as many pupils, so 900 pupils at the two schools combined are girls.

The average absenteeism of girls is 7%. We know that 900 of the 1100 girls have an average absenteeism rate of 6%. Let the average absenteeism rate of girls at Hurlington Academy be r. Then 900 x 0.06 +200r = 0.07x1100. Hence 54+200r=77. 77-54 = 200r. 23/200 = r. r=0.115. Hence, the rate of absenteeism amongst girls at Hurlington Academy is 11.5%

Question 20: D

She needs to print 400 x 2 = 800 double sided A4 sheets, which will cost 0.01 x 2 x 1.5 = £0.03 each. Hence the total cost of this is 800 x 0.03 = £24. She also needs to print 1500 single sided A5 sheets, costing £0.01 each, giving a total of 1500 x 0.01 = £15. Hence the total cost is £39.

Question 21: B

We can tell the amounts for the green party and the blue party are both 1/3 of the total, and that the amount for the red party is 1/4 of the total. Hence 1/12 is left, so the amount for the yellow party must be 1/12. Hence the red party have 3 times the intended vote of the yellow party.

Question 22: E

In Rovers' first 3 games, they have scored 1 goal and had 8 goals scored against them. In total they scored 1 goal and had 10 goals scored against them, so they must have lost their last game against United 2-0. In City's first 3 games, they scored 7 goals and had 3 goals scored against them. In total they scored 10 goals and had 4 goals scored against them, so they must have won their game against United 3-1. Hence the answer is E.

Question 23: G

The replacement of dying, damaged, and lost cells, the growth of the embryonic cell to a multi-cellular organism, and asexual reproduction are the three main reasons why cells divide through mitosis.

Question 24: E

Blood pressure in the aorta is the highest of any vessel in the body, as blood has just been ejected from the left ventricle to go to the body. The pressure in the left ventricle (and hence the Aorta) is higher than that in the right ventricle (and hence the Pulmonary Artery) because the pressure must be sufficient to pump to the entire body, rather than just the lungs.

Question 25: C

A sensory receptor (1) senses the heat of the pan. This information is passed down the sensory neurone (2) through a relay neurone to the motor neurone (4), which then causes the muscle (5) to contract, pulling the finger away.

Question 26: C

The receptor is directly coupled to the sensory neurone, so the communication here is electrical. All information between neurones passes via synapses, which use neurotransmitters to convey the information chemically. This occurs between the sensory neurone and the relay neurone, and between the relay neurone and the motor neurone. Therefore, the answer is C).

Question 27: C

Increasing the concentration of the reactants (not products) would affect reaction rate, which can be monitored by measuring the gas volume released (proportional to molar concentration). This is the reaction for photosynthesis, which does not occur spontaneously and is endothermic.

Question 28: D

Taking the diseased allele to be X^D and X as the normal allele, we can model the scenario in the Punnett square below:

		Carrier Mother	
		X^D	X
Diseased Father	X^D	$X^D X^D$	$X^D X$
	Y	$X^D Y$	XY

Boys are XY and girls are XX. 50% of the boys produced would have DMD. So the probability that both boys would have the disease is 0.5 x 0.5 = 0.25

Question 29: E

We can see from the Punnett square that the probability of having a girl with DMD is 25% ($X^D X^D$). The probability that both are girls with DMD is 0.25 x 0.25 = 0.125.

Question 30: B

All of the following statements are examples of natural selection, except for the breeding of horses. Breeding and animal husbandry are notable methods of artificial selection, which are brought about by humans.

Question 31: C

Chemical reactions take place in the cytoplasm, and the mitochondrion is the site for aerobic respiration releasing energy. The lack of a cell wall means that this is an animal cell.

Question 32: D

White blood cells can engulf/phagocytose pathogens in order to kill them. CO_2 is transported in the plasma, not in blood cells.

Question 33: C

Enzymes create a stable environment to stabilise the transition state. Enzymes do not distort substrates. Enzymes generally have little effect on temperature directly. Lastly, they are able to provide alternative pathways for reactions to occur.

Question 34: C

A negative feedback system seeks to minimise changes in a system by modulating the response in accordance with the error that's generated. Salivating before a meal is an example of a feed-forward system (i.e. salivating is an anticipatory response). Throwing a dart does not involve any feedback (during the action). pH and blood pressure are both important homeostatic variables that are controlled via powerful negative feedback mechanisms, e.g. massive haemorrhage leads to compensatory tachycardia.

Question 35: A

One of the major functions of white blood cells is to defend the body against bacterial and fungal infections. They can kill pathogens by engulfing them and also use antibodies to help them recognise pathogens. Antibodies are produced by white blood cells.

Question 36: B

The CV system does indeed transport nutrients and hormones. It also increases blood flow to exercising muscles (via differential vasodilatation) and also helps with thermoregulation (e.g. vasoconstriction in response to cold). The respiratory system is responsible for oxygenating blood.

Question 37: C

Adrenaline always increases heart rate and is almost always released during sympathetic responses. It travels primarily in the blood and affects multiple organ systems. It is also a potent vasoconstrictor.

Question 38: B

Protein synthesis occurs in the cytoplasm. Proteins are usually coded by several amino acids. Red blood cells lack a nucleus and, therefore, the DNA to create new proteins. Protein synthesis is a key part of mitosis, as it allows the parent cell to grow prior to division.

Question 39: F

Remember that most enzymes work better in neutral environments (amylase works even better at slightly alkaline pH). Thus, adding sodium bicarbonate will increase the pH and hence increase the rate of activity. Adding carbohydrate will have no effect, as the enzyme is already saturated. Adding amylase will increase the amount of carbohydrate that can be converted per unit time. Increasing the temperature to $100°$ C will denature the enzyme and reduce the rate.

Question 40: E

Taking the normal allele to be C and the diseased allele to be c, one can model the scenario with the following Punnett square:

		Carrier Mother	
		C	c
Diseased Father	c	Cc	cc
	c	Cc	cc

The gender of the children is irrelevant as the inheritance is autosomal recessive, but we see that all children produced would inherit at least one diseased allele.

Question 41: A

This is an example of an addition reaction: the chloride and hydrogen atoms are added at the unsaturated bond of the but-2-ene, which is between the 2nd and the 3rd C-atom. If you're unsure about this type of question draw it out and the answer will be obvious.

Question 42: C

The electrolysis reaction for brine is: $2\,NaCl\ +\ 2\,H_2O\ =\ 2\,NaOH\ +\ H_2\ +\ Cl_2$
Thus, keeping in mind the stoichiometry of the given equation, the solution must be C.

Question 43: A

If the two isotopes were in equal abundance, the A_r would be 77, half-way between the two isotope masses (the average). The A_r is 76.5 (a weighted average), one quarter of the way between the isotopes, so there must be three times as much of the lighter isotope to move the A_r closer to its mass of 76 ($0.75\times76 + 0.25\times78 = 76.5$).

Though there is more of ^{76}X than ^{78}X, this does not necessarily imply that ^{78}X is lost through decay, as opposed to naturally less abundant from the beginning, so there is no way to know the relative stability of the isotopes.

Question 44: C

Increasing the concentration of the reactants (not products) would affect reaction rate, which can be monitored by measuring the gas volume released (proportional to molar concentration). This is the reaction for photosynthesis, which does not occur spontaneously and is endothermic.

Question 45: H

Most polymers are made up of alkenes, which are unsaturated molecules. Polymerisation does not release water, as it is an addition reaction. Depending on the monomer molecule, polymers can take a variety of shapes.

Question 46: B

The equation for the reaction is: $Zn + CuSO_4 \rightarrow ZnSO_4 + Cu$

Assign oxidation numbers for each element:

For Zn: $Zn = 0$

For $CuSO_4$: $Cu = +2$; $S = +6$; $O = -2$

For $ZnSO_4$: $Zn = +2$; $S = +6$; $O = -2$

For Cu: $Cu = 0$

With these oxidation numbers, we can see that Zn was oxidized and Cu in $CuSO_4$ was reduced. Thus, Zn acted as the reducing agent and Cu in $CuSO_4$ is the oxidizing agent.

Question 47: B

Acids are proton donors which only exist in aqueous solution, which is a liquid state. Strong acids are fully ionised in solution and the reaction between an acid and a base $\rightarrow$ salt + water.

The pH of weak acids is usually between 4 and 6.

Question 48: G

Let x be the relative abundance of Z^6 and y the relative abundance of Z^8.

The average atomic mass takes the abundances of all 3 isotopes into account.

Thus, (Abundance of Z^5)(Mass Z^5) + (Abundance of Z^6)(Mass Z^6) + (Abundance of Z^8)(Mass Z^8) = 7

Therefore: $(5 \times 0.2) + 6x + 8y = 7$

So: $6x + 8y = 6$

Divide by two to give: $3x + 4y = 3$

The abundances of all isotopes = 100% = 1

This gives: $0.2 + x + y = 1$

Solve the two equations simultaneously:

$y = 0.8 - x$

$3x + 4(0.8 - x) = 3$

$3x + 3.2 - 4x = 3$

Therefore, $x = 0.2$

$y = 0.8 - 0.2 = 0.6$

Thus, the overall abundances are $Z^5 = 20\%$, $Z^6 = 20\%$ and $Z^8 = 60\%$. Therefore, all the statements are correct.

Question 49: A

If a metal is more reactive than hydrogen, a displacement reaction will occur resulting in the formation of a salt with the metal cation and hydrogen.

Question 50: B

$6\ FeSO_4 + K_2Cr_2O_7 + 7\ H_2SO_4 \rightarrow 3\ (Fe)_2(SO_4)_3 + Cr_2(SO_4)_3 + K_2SO_4 + 7\ H_2O$

In order to save time, you have to quickly eliminate options (rather than try every combination out).

The quickest way is to do this is algebraically:

For Potassium:

$2b = 2e = 2f$

Therefore, $b = f$.

Option F does not fulfil $b = e = f$.

For Iron:

$a = 2d$

Options C, D and E don't fulfil $a = 2d$.

For Hydrogen:

$2c = 2g$

Therefore, $c = g$.

Option A does not fulfil $c = g$.

This leaves option B as the answer.

Question 51: E

Atoms are electrically neutral. Ions have different numbers of electrons when compared to atoms of the same element. Protons provide just under 50% of an atom's mass, the other 50% is provided by neutrons. Isotopes don't exhibit significantly different kinetics. Protons do indeed repel each other in the nucleus (which is one reason why neutrons are needed: to reduce the electrical charge density).

Question 52: B

The noble gasses are extremely useful, e.g. helium in blimps, neon signs, argon in bulbs. They are colourless and odourless and have no valence electrons. As with the rest of the periodic table, boiling point increases as you progress down the group (because of increased Van der Waals forces). Helium is the most abundant noble gas (and indeed the 2nd most abundant element in the universe).

Question 53: F

This question will discriminate between students who spot short-cuts built into questions to save valuable time and those that simply dive straight in without appraising the question.

The key here is that due to the conservation of energy, all the gravitational potential energy, mgh, at the top of the ramp will be converted to kinetic energy, ½mv², at the bottom.
Thus, we can calculate the final velocity using the following: mgh = ½mv²
Note that the mass cancels so there is no need to use the density and volume information in order to calculate mass.
Hence we get: 2gh = v²
V² = 2 x 10 x 20 = 400
Therefore, v = 20 ms⁻¹

Question 54: D

Waves do not transfer mass, but their net neutral motions can interfere with each other to cause standing waves or other interference patterns. The energy of a wave depends on frequency, so waves have many different energies. Gamma rays have the highest energy for light, while visible light is lower in energy.

Question 55: A

Multiply by the denominator to give: $(7x + 10) = (3z^2 + 2)(9x + 5)$
Partially expand brackets on right side: $(7x + 10) = 9x(3z^2 + 2) + 5(3z^2 + 2)$
Take x terms across to left side: $7x - 9x(3z^2 + 2) = 5(3z^2 + 2) - 10$
Take x outside the brackets: $x[7 - 9(3z^2 + 2)] = 5(3z^2 + 2) - 10$

Thus: $x = \frac{5(3z^2 + 2) - 10}{7 - 9(3z^2 + 2)}$

Simplify to give: $x = \frac{(15z^2)}{[7 - 9(3z^2 + 2)]}$

Question 56: B

An alpha particle is a helium nucleus consisting of 2 protons and 2 neutrons. An alpha decay therefore reduces the atomic (proton) number by 2 and the mass number by 4. After a single alpha decay, the resulting proton number is 88 and the resulting mass number is 184. As this then splits in to two, the resulting element has a proton number of 44 and a mass number of 92. Gamma radiation does not alter the subatomic particle make-up of an atom.

Question 57: B

The shortest distance between points A and B is a direct line. Using Pythagoras:
The diagonal of a sports field $= \sqrt{40^2 + 30^2} = \sqrt{1,600 + 900} = \sqrt{2,500} = 50$.
The diagonal between the sports fields $= \sqrt{4^2 + 3^2} = \sqrt{16 + 9} = \sqrt{25} = 5$.
Thus, the shortest distance between A and B $= 50 + 5 + 50 = 105\,m$.

Question 58: C

Let $y = 1.25 \times 10^8$; this is not necessary, but helpful, as the question can then be expressed as: $\frac{100y + 10y}{2y} = \frac{110y}{2y} = 55$

Question 59: A

Equate y to give:

$2x - 1 = x^2 - 1$

$\rightarrow x^2 - 2x = 0$

$\rightarrow x(x - 2) = 0$

Thus, x = 2 and x = 0

There is no need to substitute back to get the y values as only option A satisfies the x values.

Question 60: B

The ruler and the cruise ship look to be the same size because their edges are in line with Tim's line of sight. His eyes form the apex of two similar triangles. All the sides of two similar triangles are in the same ratio since the angles are the same, therefore:

$\frac{0.3m}{X m} = \frac{1 m}{1 m + 999 m}$

Thus, $X m = 1000 m \times \frac{0.3 m}{1 m}$

$1000 \times 0.3 = 300 m$

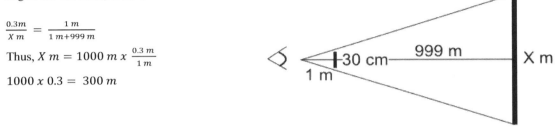

END OF PAPER

Mock Paper G Answers

Question 1: B
The Kabbalah is an esoteric Jewish system. Popular will celebrities, Madonna, among others, is an adherent.

Question 2: B
Pompeii was destroyed by the eruption, but was perfectly preserved by the ash, and is now our main source of knowledge about the lives of everyday Romans. Herculaneum, the neighbouring city to Pompeii was also destroyed.

Question 3: A
Guernica was bombed by the Nazis at the request of the fascist party of Spain, led by Francisco Franco, during the Spanish civil war.

Question 4: C
A Dinosaur is a 'terrible lizard' in Greek.

Question 5: C
The nine muses, who inspired Greek artists and writers in different fields of study.

Question 6: B
Robert Mugabe was finally arrested by the army at the age of 93.

Question 7: C

Martin Luther was one of the first protestant reformers, and wrote a list of 95 issues he had with the catholic church, including the sale of indulgences.

Question 8: B
In the wake of the many atrocities in WWII the United nations set out to provide a concrete list of human rights which should not be violated.

Question 9: C
Ptolemy was a mathematician and astronomer. Ptolemy's model of the solar system had been in use since the 2nd century AD and rarely questioned, it out the earth at the centre of the solar system.

Question 10: A
The Large hadron collider is so-called because its job is to smash atoms together at incredibly high speed and observe what is produced by the collision.

Question 11: D
The Uffizi in Florence has an enormous collection of Renaissance paintings, a large percent of which were painted by people who lived or worked there. The Galleria D'ell Academia nearby is mostly renaissance sculpture.

Question 12: C
The Challenger Space Shuttle exploded while trying to leave the Earth's atmosphere.

Question 13: C

B is completely irrelevant to what the manager is saying, so is incorrect. A and E are also incorrect as the manager is simply talking about ticket sales. He has not mentioned anything about the relevant popularity of folk music, or how much the band should value profit. D is incorrect as the manager is simply saying that the band will have higher ticket sales in France than in Germany, so other countries are not relevant. C is correct as Germany could still have higher ticket sales for folk music than France despite the recent changes in ticket sales.

Question 14: E

A is completely irrelevant to John's conclusions, as the speed of travel has no effect on the train's destination. D is also irrelevant as other destinations from King's Cross station also bear no effect on John's conclusion. Meanwhile, B is incorrect as John's conclusions refer to travelling to Edinburgh by train, so the possibility of travelling by aeroplane has no effect. C is not an assumption because John's conclusion is in the present tense, referring to journeys made at the moment, so future developments have no effect. E is an assumption John has made. Only two other stations in London have been mentioned. At no point has it been mentioned that there are no other stations in London that John could travel from.

Question 15: E

We can work out the code for each number and see which one equals 3.
The code for A is (3x4) = 12, divided by 6 = 2, minus 1 = 1
The code for B is (9x8) = 72, divided by 6 = 12, minus 4 = 8
The code for C is (5x4) = 20, divided by 2 = 10, minus 3 = 7
The code for D is (7x8) = 56, divided by 4 = 14, minus 8 = 6
The code for E is (6x8) = 48, divided by 4 = 12, minus 9 = 3
Therefore the pin number with the code 3 is E, 6839.

Question 16: E

We can calculate all the rental yields as follows:
House A: (700x12)/168000 = 0.05
House B: (40x125x4)/200000 = 20000/200000 = 0.10
House C: (600*12)/144000 = 7200/144000 = 0.05
House D: (2000*12)/240000 = 24000/240000 = 0.10
House E: (200*52)/100000 = 10400/100000. We can see by observation that this is > 0.1 as 10000/100000 would equal 0.1, therefore there is no need to work this out to be able to say that this is the house with the highest yield.

Question 17: C

The question says that Shaniqua plays in the square which will stop Summer being able to win straight away, so Shaniqua must play in 4. Summer then needs to play in a square where there will be 2 different options to make a line on the turn afterwards, so that Shaniqua cannot block both of them. If Summer plays in 1, she can make a line by playing in either 5 or 6 the next turn, so Shaniqua cannot stop her winning. If Summer plays in 2, she cannot make a line on the next turn at all. If Summer plays in 3, she can only make a line by playing in 6 the next turn and so Shaniqua can stop her. If Summer plays in 5, she can only make a line by playing in 5 the next turn and so Shaniqua can stop her. If Summer plays in 6, she can make a line by playing in either 1 or 3 the next turn, so Shaniqua cannot stop her winning. Therefore she either needs to play in 1 or 6 to be able to be certain of winning the next time.

Question 18: B

The volume of the box with 10cm squares cut out is 10*100*100 = 100000cm^3
The volume of the box with 20cm squares cut out is 20*80*80 = 128000cm^3
The volume of the box with 30cm squares cut out is 30*60*60 = 108000cm^3
The volume of the box with 40cm squares cut out is 40*40*40 = 64000cm^3
The volume of the box with 50cm squares cut out is 50*20*20 = 20000cm^3
Therefore the biggest box is the one with the 20cm squares cut out, so the answer is B.

Question 19: A

At no point is A stated, but if aeroplanes are not a major source of carbon dioxide then it does not follow that they are largely responsible for the damage caused by global warming. Therefore, A is a valid assumption.

B and C are both stated in the question, whilst D is irrelevant to the conclusion. E, meanwhile, is stated, as the question states that *we must now seek to curb air traffic in order to save the world's remaining natural environments.*

Question 20: B

B is an underlying assumption in the Transport Minister's argument. If rural areas have plenty of passengers, her assertion that rail companies will not run many services to these areas does not follow from her reasoning. Therefore, if B is true, it strengthens the transport minister's argument.

Meanwhile, D would actually weaken the transport minister's argument, suggesting that privatisation would not lead to less service for rural areas.

C is irrelevant as the transport minister is arguing about how rural communities will be cut off by a privatised system. She is not referring to the quality or price of rail services under a publically subsidised system.

A and E are completely irrelevant points, which have no effect at all on the strength of the Transport Minister's argument.

Question 21: D

At no point does the argument state or imply that we should not be concerned about damage to the polar ice caps, or that reducing energy consumption will not reduce CO2 emissions. Therefore, B and E are incorrect.

C could be described as an assumption made in the argument and is therefore not a conclusion.

A goes beyond what the argument says. The argument does not say there are no environmental benefits to reducing energy consumption; it merely says it will not help the Polar Ice Caps. Therefore, A is incorrect and C is a valid conclusion from the argument.

Question 22: B

E is contradictory to the main conclusion of the argument.

A, C and D are all reasons which go on to support the main conclusion of the argument, which is given in B. If we accept A, C and D as true, then it follows readily that the statement given in B is true. Therefore, B is the main conclusion.

Question 23: B

Natural selection favours those who are best suited for survival – this can mean faster and stronger organisms, but not always. For example, snails are pervasive, despite being weak and slow. Variation can arise due to both genetic and environmental components.

Question 24: D

The enzyme amylase catalyses the breakdown of starch into sugars in the mouth (1) and the small intestine (5).

Question 25: E

Whilst there is some enzymatic digestion in 1 and 3, the vast majority occurs in the small intestine (5). The liver facilitates digestion via the production of bile, and the large intestine is primarily responsible for the absorption of water.

Question 26: A
Replotting the genetic diagram with genotype information produces the diagram:

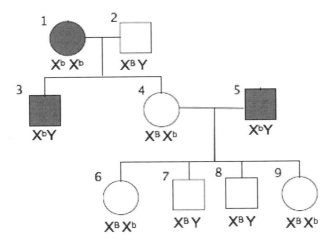

If squares were female, all of 5's circular male offspring would be affected. Circles must be females, so 1 must be homozygous recessive.

Question 27: D
The genotype of a heterozygote female is be $X^B X^b$, and the genotype of 8 is $X^B Y$. Plotting the information in a Punnett square:

		Female Heterozygote	
		X^B	X^b
Individual 8 (Unaffected Male)	X^B	$X^B X^B$	$X^B X^b$
	Y	$X^B Y$	$X^b Y$

The progeny produced are 25% $X^B X^B$ (homozygous normal female), 25% $X^B X^b$ (heterozygous carrier female), 25% $X^B Y$ (normal male) and 25% $X^b Y$ (affected male). So the chance of producing a colour blind boy is 25%.

Question 28: A
Urine passes from the kidney into the ureter and is then stored in the bladder. It is finally released through the urethra.

Question 29: B
As the known parent has both recessive genotypes, it can only have the gametes, y and t. The next generation has a phenotypic ratio of 1:1:1:1. As both recessive and dominant traits are present in the progeny, the unknown parent's genotype must contain both the recessive and dominant alleles. Hence the unknown parent's genotype must be YyTt as this would produce the gamete combinations of YT, Yt, yT and yt, which when combined with the known yt gametes would result in YyTt, Yytt, yyTt and yytt in equal ratios.

Question 30: D
The possible genotypes are: YYTT (yellow, tall), YyTT (yellow, tall), yyTT (green, tall), YYTt (yellow, tall), YYtt (yellow, short), YyTt (yellow, tall) Yytt (yellow, short), yyTt (green, tall), yytt (green, short). Thus, 9 different genotypes and 4 different phenotypes are possible.

Question 31: D

Whilst getting vitamins, killing bacteria, protein synthesis, and maintaining cellular pH and temperature are all important processes that require a blood supply, the MOST important reason for having a blood supply is the delivery of oxygen and removal of CO_2. This allows aerobic respiration to take place, which produces energy for all of the cell's metabolic processes. None of these processes can be sustained for a meaningful period of time without the energy made available from respiration.

Question 32: A

Insulin works to decrease blood glucose levels. Glucagon causes blood glucose levels to increase; glycogen is a carbohydrate. Adrenaline works to increase heart rate.

Question 33: A

The left side of the heart contains oxygenated blood from the lungs which will be pumped to the body. The right side of the heart contains deoxygenated blood from the body to be pumped to the lungs.

Question 34: A

Since Individual 1 is homozygous normal, and individual 5 is heterozygous and affected, the disease must be dominant. Since males only have one X-chromosome, they cannot be carriers for X-linked conditions. If Nafram syndrome was X-linked, then parents 5 and 6 would produce sons who always have no disease and daughters that always do. As this is not the case shown in individuals 7-10, the disease must be autosomal dominant.

Question 35: C

We know that the inheritance of Nafram syndrome is autosomal dominant, so using N to mean a diseased allele and n to mean a normal allele, 5, 7 and 8 must be Nn because they have an unaffected parent. 2 is also Nn, as if it was NN all its progeny would be Nn and so affected by the disease, which is not the case, as 3 and 4 are unaffected.

Question 36: A

Since 6 is disease free, his genotype must be nn. Thus, neither of 6's parents could be NN, as otherwise 6 would have at least one diseased allele.

Question 37: F

All of the organs listed have endocrine functions. The thyroid produces thyroid hormone. The ovary produces oestrogen. The pancreas secretes glucagon and insulin. The adrenal gland secretes adrenaline. The testes produce testosterone.

Question 38: F

Deoxygenated blood from the body flows through the inferior vena cava to the right atrium where it flows to the right ventricle to be pumped via the pulmonary artery to the lungs where it is oxygenated. It then returns to the heart via the pulmonary vein into the left atrium into the left ventricle where it is pumped to the body via the aorta.

Question 39: E

During inspiration, the pressure in the lungs decreases as the diaphragm contracts, increasing the volume of the lungs. The intercostal muscles contract in inspiration, lifting the rib cage.

Question 40: D

The hypothalamus is the site of central thermoreceptors. A decrease in environmental temperature decreases sweat secretion and causes cutaneous vasoconstriction to minimise heat loss from the blood.

Question 41: H

Chloride is oxidised during this process to form Cl_2. Although the first part of 2) is correct, H_2O is required to dissolve the NaCl (not H_2 which is a product of the reaction). NaOH is a strong base.

Question 42: B

This is an example of an addition reaction, the fluorine and hydrogen atoms are added at the unsaturated bond. If you're unsure about this type of question draw it out and the answer will be obvious.

Question 43: A

The hydrogen halide binds to the alkene's unsaturated double bond. This results in a fully saturated product that consists purely of covalent bonds.

Question 44: F

All of the above are true. Every mole of gas occupies the same volume. The left side therefore occupies 4 volumes, and the right side occupies 2 volumes. Increasing pressure will favour the lower volume side, and the equilibrium will shift right to produce ammonia and decrease the overall volume that the products and reactants occupy. If more N_2 gas is added, equilibrium will shift to react away this gas and lower the concentration again, with the result that more ammonia will be formed.

Question 45: E

Sodium is element 11 on the periodic table, a group 1 element, so has electron configuration: 2, 8, 1. It forms a metallic bond with other sodium atoms. Chlorine is element 17 in group 7, so has 17 electrons and 7 valence electrons, giving configuration: 2, 8, 7. Chlorine forms the covalent gas Cl_2, sharing one electron for a full valence shell.

Salt (NaCl) is an ionic compound, where sodium gives its single valence electron to chlorine so both atoms have full outer electron shells (8 electrons, so 2, 8:2, 8, 8).

Question 46: A

The polymerisation reaction opens the double bond between the two C atoms to allow the formation of a long chain of monomers.

Question 47: C

Assume total mass of molecule is 100g. Therefore, it contains 70.6g carbon, 5.9g hydrogen and 23.5g oxygen. Now, calculate the number of moles of each element using $Moles = \frac{Mass}{Molar\ Mass}$

$Moles\ of\ Carbon = \frac{70.6}{12} \approx 6$

$Moles\ of\ Hydrogen = \frac{5.9}{1} \approx 6$

$Moles\ of\ Oxygen = \frac{23.5}{16} \approx 1.5$

Therefore, the molar ratios give an empirical formula of $C_6H_6O_{1.5} = C_4H_4O$.
Molar mass of the empirical formula = (4 x 12) + (4 x 1) + 16 = 68.
Molar mass of chemical formula = 136. Therefore, the chemical formula = $C_8H_8O_2$.

Question 48: D

Alkenes can be hydrogenated (i.e. reduced) to alkanes. Aromatic compounds are commonly written as cyclic alkenes, but their properties differ from those of alkenes. Therefore alkenes and aromatic compounds do not belong to the same chemical class.

Question 49: A

Transition metals form multiple stable ions which may have many different colours (e.g. green Fe^{2+} and brown Fe^{3+}). They usually form ionic bonds and are commonly used as catalysts (e.g. iron in the Haber process, Nickel in alkene hydrogenation). They are excellent conductors of electricity and are known as the d-block elements.

Question 50: A

The average atomic mass takes the abundances of both isotopes into account:

(Abundance of Cl^{35})(Mass Cl^{35}) + (Abundance of Cl^{37})(Mass Cl^{37}) = 35.453

34.969(Abundance of Cl^{35}) + 36.966(Abundance of Cl^{37}) = 35.453

The abundances of both isotopes = 100% = 1

I.e. abundance of Cl^{35} + abundance of Cl^{37} = 1

Therefore: $x + y = 1$ which can be rearranged to give: $y = 1 - x$

Therefore: $x + (1 - x) = 1$.

$34.969x + 36.966(1-x) = 35.453$

$x = 0.758$

$1 - x = 0.242$

Therefore, Cl^{35} is 3 times more abundant than Cl^{37}.

Note that you could approximate the values here to arrive at the solution even quicker, e.g. 34.969 → 35, 36.966 → 37 and 35.453 → 35.5

Question 51: B

$2Na + 2H_2O \rightarrow 2NaOH + H_2$

8000 cm^3 = 8 dm^3 = ⅓ moles of H_2

2 moles of Na react completely to form 1 mole of H_2.

Therefore, ⅔ moles of Na must have reacted to produce ⅓ moles of Hydrogen. ⅔ x 23g per mole = 15.3g.

% Purity of sample $= \frac{15.3}{20}$ x 100 = 76.5%

Question 52: B

$S + 6 HNO_3 \rightarrow H_2SO_4 + 6 NO_2 + 2 H_2O$

In order to save time, you have to quickly eliminate options (rather than try every combination out).

The quickest way to do this is algebraically:

For Hydrogen:

$b = 2c + 2e$

Options A, C, D, E and F don't fulfil $b = 2c + 2e$.

This leaves options B as the only possible answer.

Note how quickly we were able to get the correct answer here by choosing an element that appears in 3 molecules (as opposed to Sulphur or Nitrogen which only appear in 2).

Question 53: D

The energy in a nuclear bomb comes from $E = mc^2$. When two nuclei fuse, the combined mass is slightly smaller than the two individual nuclei, and the mass lost is converted to energy according to Einstein's equation. Fusion releases much more energy than fission, as in the sun, and humans cannot harness this energy yet. Uncontrolled fission causes the explosion in an atom bomb and is created by a neutron-induced chain reaction. In power plants these neutrons are tightly controlled, so as not to overload the reactors and cause an explosion.

Question 54: B

$$\left(\frac{T}{4\pi}\right)^2 = \frac{l(M + 3m)}{3g(M + 2m)}$$

$$\frac{T^2}{16\pi^2} \times \frac{3g}{l} = \frac{M + 3m}{M + 2m}$$

$$3gT^2(M + 2m) = 16l\pi^2(M + 3m)$$

$$3gT^2M + 6gT^2m = 16l\pi^2M + 48l\pi^2m$$

$$6gT^2m - 48l\pi^2m = 16l\pi^2M - 3gT^2M$$

$$m(6gT^2 - 48l\pi^2) = 16l\pi^2M - 3gT^2M$$

$$m = \frac{16l\pi^2M - 3gT^2M}{6gT^2 - 48l\pi^2}$$

Question 55: B
The mean is the sum of all the numbers in the set divided by the number of members in the set. The sum of all the numbers in the original set must be: 11 numbers x mean of 6 = 66. The sum of all the numbers once two are removed must then be: 9 numbers x mean of 5 = 45. Thus any two numbers which sum to 66 − 45 = 21 could have been removed from the set.

Question 56: B
R of series circuit= R + R = 2R

$$R \text{ parallel} = \frac{1}{\frac{1}{R}+\frac{1}{R}} = \frac{1}{\frac{2}{R}} = \frac{R}{2}$$

Thus, the parallel circuit has a smaller resistance than the series circuit.
Since $I = \frac{V}{R}$, the parallel circuit will have a greater current than the series.

Question 57: B
Let $y = 3.4 \times 10^{10}$; this is not necessary, but helpful, as the question can then be expressed as:
$$\frac{10y + y}{200y} = \frac{11y}{200y} = \frac{11}{200} = \frac{5.5}{100}$$
$$= 5.5 \times 10^{-2}$$

Question 58: E
From the rules of angles made by intersections with parallel lines, all of the angles marked with the same letter are equal. There is no way to find if d = 90°, only that b + d = c = 180° − a = 135°, so b is unknown.

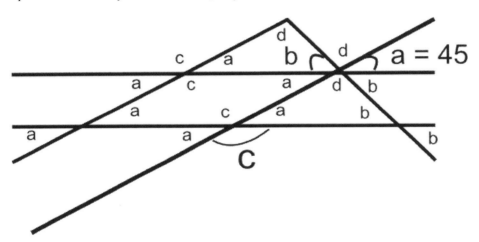

Question 59: B

During electrolysis a current is used to draw charged ions to electrodes. The anode is positively charged and draws anions like sulphate, and the cathode is negatively charged and attracts positively charged cations like copper. For electrolysis to work well, the electrodes need to keep their positive or negative charge. If an alternating AC-current was used, the anode and cathode would repeatedly switch places, and the ions would make no net movement toward either electrode.

Question 60: C

Transform all numbers into fractions then follow the order of operations to simplify. Move the surds next to each other and evaluate systematically:

$$= \left(\left(\frac{6}{8} \times \frac{7}{3}\right) \div \left(\frac{7}{5} \times \frac{2}{6}\right)\right) \times \frac{4}{10} \times \frac{15}{100} \times \frac{5}{100} \times \frac{5}{25} \times \pi \times \left(\sqrt{e^2}\right) \times e\pi^{-1}$$

$$= \left(\frac{42}{24} \div \frac{14}{30}\right) \times \frac{4 \times 3 \times 25}{10 \times 20 \times 100 \times 25} \times \pi \times \pi^{-1} \times e^{-1} \times e$$

$$= \left(\frac{21}{12} \div \frac{7}{15}\right) \times \frac{12}{200 \times 100} \times \frac{\pi}{\pi} \times \frac{e}{e}$$

$$= \left(\frac{21}{12} \times \frac{15}{7}\right) \times \frac{3}{50 \times 100}$$

$$= \frac{45}{12} \times \frac{3}{5000}$$

$$= \frac{9}{4} \times \frac{1}{1000}$$

$$= \frac{9}{4000}$$

END OF PAPER

Mock Paper H Answers

Question 1: D
The Sagrada Familia, is the Cathedral in Barcelona designed by Gaudi. It is typical for cathedrals to take hundreds of years to build.

Question 2: D
Proverbs, Ecclesiastes and psalms are all examples of Songs and Wisdom literature from the Bible, and contain some beautiful poetry and musing on life.

Question 3: C
The Mau Mau uprising was in Kenya. By the 1950's India had already gained it's independence, Jamaica gained their independence peacefully in 1962, and Zimbabwe in 1980. South Africa was a Dutch colony.

Question 4: A
The Social Contract an important text at the time of the French Revolution. The quote is frequently confused with the Karl Marx statement that 'You have nothing to lose but your chains!' from the Communist manifesto.

Question 5: B
The Latin name for silver is Argentum, hence Argentina.

Question 6: E
Lebanon, which is famous around the world for its cedar trees.

Question 7: B
Better known for his theories about dreams and the sex drive, Sigmund Freud also postulated a death drive, or human drive towards destruction.

Question 8: D
Before the Ottoman conquest, Istanbul was Constantinople, the capital of the Byzantine empire, and before that it was a Greek city state called Byzantium.

Question 9: D
Bootlegging was the smuggling of alcohol. The word comes from the American civil war, when soldiers smuggled alcohol in their boots and trousers.

Question 10: A
They all died in office. Although both Kennedy and McKinley were assassinated. Roosevelt died of a brain haemorrhage a few months into his fourth term of office.

Question 11: D
Sylvia Plath wrote the novel about her struggles with depression whilst living and working in New York City.

Question 12: B
A Stradivarius is a type of violin made by the Stradivari family in Italy. Some of their violins, from their heyday period in the 18th century, are worth millions of dollars.

Question 13: A
In this question we are looking at what cannot be reliably concluded from the passage. B and E conclude the state of a substance is not dependent on its chemical properties. C and D discuss how combining two substances can produce a new substance with very different physical properties. The passage refers to how the chemistry of a compound does not necessarily affect the physical properties of that compound. Thus, the answer must be A, which claims the chemical composition of a compound influences its physical nature.

Question 14: E

In this question we are looking at what can be reliably concluded from the passage. The passage is referring to products being made from similar parts; it is the way in which these parts are arranged that actually determines the final product. Thus, B cannot be right. D is also not correct, as there is no mention of protoplasm being the building block for life. E is the correct answer therefore.

Question 15: D

With these questions it is easiest to start at the end of the question and work backwards. The day two days before Monday is Saturday. The day immediately after that is Sunday. The day that comes four days after Sunday is Thursday, and two days after that is Saturday. Thus, the answer is D.

Question 16: E

In order to work out this question, we need to make some simultaneous equations to relate John and Michael's money. If the amount of money John has at the start is J, and the amount that Michael has is M, we get the following equations:

$J - 20 = 2(M + 20)$ and $J + 5 = 5(M - 5)$, which is simplified to:

$J = 2M + 60$ and $J = 5M - 30$.

Substituting in, to work out M gives:

$2M + 60 = 5M - 30$, thus $3M = 90$ and $M = 30$.

Substituting in $M = 30$ to one of the equations gives:

$J = 60 + 60 = 120$.

Thus, $J + M = 150$, so the answer is E.

Question 17: E

In this question we want a summary of the passage. This passage refers to the use of fire in civilisations to create light. Through the passage it talks about the evolution of the use of fire, finishing with a reference to gas lamps in the street. Thus a good conclusion will refer to how the use of fire has changed over time, but also how lighting one's home is a key factor of civilisation. The answer must therefore be E, which discusses the evolution of fire use and also its importance in civilisation.

Question 18: C

In this question we are looking at what can be reliably concluded from the passage. The passage does not tell us exactly how phosphorous was discovered, but we know that it was not Wilhelm Homberg who discovered it, thus A, B and D cannot be correct. 1669 is not in the 18th century thus E is also false. The passage describes how the element phosphorous was discovered by accident, by a man of low social status. Therefore, C is the only correct answer.

Question 19: D

For this question refer to the times in minutes, rather than hours, so 3pm is 180 minutes. x is the number of minutes past noon that we are trying to find. Therefore $x + 28$ will give the same amount of minutes past noon as $180 - 3x$.

$x + 28 = 180 - 3x$

$4x = 152$

$x = 38$, thus the answer is D.

Question 20: B

In this question we are trying to find a suitable conclusion to the passage. A and E are completely irrelevant to the passage. C is incorrect as wings only attach to the posterior two segments of the insect's body. While D is correct, the legs are not referenced as being the most important part of the insect's body. Thus the answer must be B, which states the wings are the most dominant part of the body.

Question 21: D
For John: 56/64 x 100 = 87.5% or 7/8
For Mary: 24/36 x 100 = 66.7% or 2/3
Therefore we need to work out 7/8 – 2/3
21/24 – 16/24 = 5/24. Multiply by 100 to get the actual percentage:
500/24 = 125/6, thus the answer is D.

Question 22: A
To calculate this one needs to find the lowest common multiple of both 73 and 104, and then add that value to 2007. The lowest common multiple of 73 and 104 is 7592, which when added to 2007 gives 9559AD.

Question 23: A
HCO_3^- is an alkaline substance and a vital component of the physiological buffering system. If the pH of the blood drops below 7, the bicarbonate molecule will accept a H^+ whereas if the pH increase, it will release H^+, thus HCO_3^- is an alkali.

Question 24: D
The diaphragm is crucial to breathing as during inhalation it contracts and expands the chest space, along with the intercostal muscles which draw the ribs upwards and outwards, effectively lowering the pressure within the thoracic cavity and drawing air into the lungs. During exhalation all the muscles relax which lets the ribs drop downwards and inwards and the diaphragm balloons upwards into the chest space. This increases the pressure within the thoracic cavity which forces air out of the lungs.

Question 25: E
Some students may think that the arteries carry oxygenated blood from the mother to the foetus and that the vein carries the deoxygenated blood from the foetus to the mother, but it is important to remember that arteries always carry blood to the heart (in this case the mother's) and veins always travel away from the heart. A prime example of this is the pulmonary system, as like the foetal-mother system, the pulmonary arteries carry deoxygenated blood to the lungs away from the heart and the pulmonary veins carry oxygenated blood back to the heart.

Question 26: H
The kidneys are involved in ultrafiltration as they filter all of the blood in the body of toxins/waste products from metabolic reactions. The waste is released as urine via the bladder. Some of the water is filtered out then reabsorbed by the kidney, especially when the body is dehydrated. Although glucose is reabsorbed by the kidney, it does not play a part in glucose regulation as that is mainly done by the pancreas by secretion of insulin and glucagon. These hormones are two of many found in the body, none of which are produced by the kidneys. There are some that are produced by the adrenal cortices that sit atop the kidneys, but these are a separate anatomical structure from the kidney.

Question 27: A
Haemophilia B is an X-linked recessive disorder which means you need two copies of the faulty genes in girls to present the phenotype associated with the disease and only one copy in males as they have XY chromosomes and are thus missing the extra X chromosome which may have carried the healthy, dominant gene. As Mike, the father of the baby girl, is not affected, we can assume that the mother carries one copy of the faulty gene herself. Thus, although the baby girl will not be affected by the condition, she may be a carrier of the gene and so, can pass it on to future generations.

Question 28: F
The first line defence of the body from invading pathogens is the skin. This is a tough keratinized layer, which is not easily broken down by bacteria. There is also flora on the skin (bacteria that live on the skin) that prevents any harmful bacteria from colonising. The next line of defence is the mucus lining the airways. It traps dirt and pathogens, to be either expelled from the body or swallowed into the gut. The next layer of defence mentioned in the answers, is hydrochloric acid found in the stomach. This has a pH of 2 and so effectively kills any pathogens that enter the body through the food. Other defences not listed include, tears (they contain lysozymes that break down the bacteria) and acidic substances by the sebaceous glands of the skin.
Some students may get confused by the antibodies. Although it is true that antibodies provide a line of defence, they are a secondary line of defence after the pathogen has got past the initial defences.

Question 29: C
Osmosis is the movement of water particles across a partially permeable membrane from an area of low concentration to an area of high concentration (of solute). It is not an active process as water can easily diffuse through bilipid layer membranes and thus does not require a specific passage.

Question 30: B
Plants also give off carbon via respiration and death. Although some of the carbon is given off, trees and plants do store carbon in their cells and thus they are known as carbon stores.

Question 31: A
Enzymes are always substrate specific as the active site is made up of a specific set of amino acids that determine which reaction the enzyme catalyses.

Question 32: D
Whilst A, B, C and E are true of the DNA code, they do not represent the property described, which is that more than one combination of codons can encode the same amino acid, e.g. Serine is coded by the sequences: TCT, TCC, TCA, TCG.

Question 33: B
The degenerate nature of the code can help to reduce the deleterious effects of point mutations. The several 3-nucleotide combinations that code for each amino acid are usually similar such that a point mutation, i.e. a substitution of one nucleotide for another, can still result in the same amino acid as the one coded for by the original sequence.

Question 34: A
The movement of carbon dioxide in the lungs and neurotransmitters in a synapse are both examples of diffusion. Glucose reabsorption is an active process, as it requires work to be done against a concentration gradient.

Question 35: F
Some enzymes contain other molecules besides protein, e.g. metal ions. Enzymes can increase rates of reaction that may result in heat gain/loss, depending on if the reaction is exothermic or endothermic. They are prone to variations in pH and are highly specific to their individual substrate.

Questions 36: E
Statements 1 and 3 are correct. Statement 2 in incorrect, as it is the 4 carbon molecule oxaloacetate that is regenerated. Oxaloacetate combines with acetyl CoA to form the 6 carbon citrate.

Question 37: B
Statement 1 and 3 are incorrect. Cyclic phosphorylation doesn't require water as no photolysis occurs, the electrons are just passed back to the chlorophyll molecule. Photolysis only occurs in PSII, because this is where the enzymes are. Statement 2 is correct, photolysis of water produces protons, which can reduce NADP.

Question 38: C
Statement 1 is incorrect as RUBISCO is an enzyme that fixes carbon dioxide to RuBP. Statement 2 is correct. 6 turns of the cyle produce 12 triose phosphate moleucles. 10 are used to regenerate RuBP, and 2 removed from the cycle to form one molecule of glucose

Question 39: F
Statement 1 is correct, sodium ions drive depolarisation and potassium ions drive repolarisation. Statement 2 is correct, as hyperpolarisation prevents the initiation of another action potential in the region that has just been depolarised, so the action potential can only travel forwards. Statement 3 is correct. As temperature increases action potentials travel faster, up to around 40°C after which the proteins start to denature. Larger diameter axons have less electrical resistance, so action potentials can travel faster.

Question 40: E
Statement 1 is correct, if too much insulin is given then the blood glucose level can fall dangerously low. Statement 2 in incorrect, adrenaline increased blood glucose to allow the body to respond to a fight-or-flight situation. Statement 3 is correct, glucagon causes glycogen to be hydrolysed into glucose (glycogenolysis), and fatty acids and amino acids to be converted into glucose (gluconeogenesis)

Question 41: C
ΔH is positive because the enthalpy of the products is higher than the enthalpy of the reactants. This also means that the reactants are less stable than the products and because it is ENDOthermic, energy is absorbed from the surroundings.

Question 42: A
There are several methods to work this out, one of which is shown below.
Mass of FeS_2 in the ore = 480 x 0.75 = 360kg
1 mole of FeS_2 = 55 + 32 + 32 = 119g → this can be rounded to 120g for ease of calculation.
Number of moles of FeS_2 in the ore = $\frac{360 \times 10^3}{120}$ = 3 x 10^3 mol
Mass of Fe = (3 x 10^3) x 55 = 165kg.
167.7kg is closest to this value.

Question 43: B
Here, it is important to remember the reactivity series.
This is important as it tells you which elements are able to displace other elements in redox reactions. In this example, Zinc is the only element above Iron in the series and thus, is the only element that would be able to displace Iron.

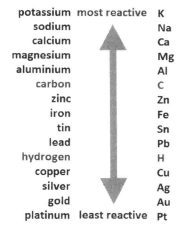

potassium most reactive	K
sodium	Na
calcium	Ca
magnesium	Mg
aluminium	Al
carbon	C
zinc	Zn
iron	Fe
tin	Sn
lead	Pb
hydrogen	H
copper	Cu
silver	Ag
gold	Au
platinum least reactive	Pt

Question 44: A
Catalysts increase the rate of reaction by providing an alternative reaction path with a lower activation energy, which means that less energy is required and so costs are reduced. The point of equilibrium, the nature of the products, and the overall energy change are unaffected by catalysts.

Question 45: A
In the diagram shown, the number at the top (73) denotes the mass number of an atom of Germanium. This is the number of protons and neutrons in the nucleus. The number at the bottom (32) is the proton number, i.e. the number of protons in the nucleus. Protons have a positive charge, neutrons have a neutral charge and electrons have a negative charge. As a stable element, Germanium must have a charge of 0 and thus the electrons and protons have to cancel out. Therefore, Germanium has 32 electrons.

Question 46: A

This is complete combustion as all of the methane is used to make water and carbon dioxide. It is an aerobic reaction as oxygen is present and needed to cause the combustion of the fuel. By increasing the carbon dioxide in the system you would either slow down or not affect the rate of combustion, but definitely would not speed it up. This also applies to removing oxygen from the system.

Question 47: A

Alkenes undergo addition reactions, such as that with hydrogen, when catalysed by nickel, whilst alkanes do not as they are already fully saturated. The C=C bond is stronger than the C-C bond, but it is not exactly twice as strong, so will not require twice the energy to break it. Both molecules are organic and will dissolve in organic solvents.

Question 48: F

Diamond is unable to conduct electricity because all the electrons are involved in covalent bonds. Graphite is insoluble in water + organic solvents. Graphite is also able to conduct electricity because there are free electrons that are not involved in covalent bonds.

Methane and Ammonia both have low melting points. Methane is not a polar molecule, so cannot conduct electricity or dissolve in water. Ammonia is polar and will dissolve in water. It can conduct electricity in aqueous form, but not as a gas.

Question 49: E

The 5 carbon atoms in this hydrocarbon make it a "pent" stem. The C=C bond makes it an alkene, and the location of this bond is the 2nd position, making the molecule pent-2-ene.

Question 50: D

Group 1 elements form positively charged ions in most reactions and therefore lose electrons. Thus, the oxidation number must increase. Their reactivity increases as the valence electrons are further away from the positively charged nucleus down group. All group one elements react spontaneously with oxygen – the less reactive ones form an oxide coating and the more reactive ones spontaneously burn.

Question 51: H

The cathode attracts positively charged ions. The cathode reduces ions and the anode oxidises ions. Electrolysis can be used to separate compounds but not mixtures (i.e. substances that are not chemically joined).

Question 52: B

Pentane, C_5H_{12}, has a total of 3 isomers. A, C and D are correctly configured. However, the 4th Carbon atom in option B has more than 4 bonds which wouldn't be possible. If you're stuck on this – draw them out!

Question 53: B

The current in a series circuit is always the same at any point in the circuit according to Kirchoff's first law which states that *at any node or junction in a circuit the sum of the current flowing into that node is equal to the current leaving that same node.* Thus current is always conserved. Since a series circuit does not have any nodes or junctions, we can assume the current is constant throughout.

The potential difference is shared between all the components of the circuit ($V_{total} = V_1 + V_2 + V_3...$). This is because the total work done on the charge by the battery must equal the total work done by the charge on the components. Resistance in a series circuit is the sum of all the individual resistances (R = R1 + R2 + R3…). The resistance of two or more resistors is bigger than the resistance of just one of the resistors on its own because the battery has to push charge through all of them.

Question 54: B

There are several steps to solving this problem. The first is to work out the area of the entire floor, minus the fish tank and the cut out corner. We can see that the length of the room is 8m and the width of the room is 4m (the sides of the cut out square are 2m). Thus the area of the entire room is **32m²**.

The cut out corner is a square with the dimension 2 x 2m. Thus the area of the cut out corner is **4m²**.

The fish tank is a circle, so its area will be πr^2. Π is taken to be 3 and thus $3 \times 1^2 = $ **3m²**.

Therefore the floor area, Bill needs to cover is $32 - (4 + 3) = $ **25m²**.

We then need to work out the area of one plank. The dimensions of this are in cm and so we need to convert to m. 1m is 100cm and so we can say that the length of the plank is 0.6m and the width is 0.1m. Thus the area is 0.6 x 0.1 = **0.06m²**.

To work out the number of planks, required, we need to divide the area of the floor space by the area of the plank. A quick way of doing this would be rounding the area of the room down to 24 and multiplying the area of the plank by 100 so it becomes 6.

24/6 = 4, then because we multiplied the area of the plank by 100, we then multiply the answer by 100 which gives us **400 planks.** The closest answer to our solution is 417, which is listed as B.

Question 55: B

Solve $y = x^2 - 3x + 4$ and $y - x = 1$ as (x,y).

Substitute the quadratic expression into the other non-quadratic. You'll get another equation.

$x + 1 = x^2 - 3x + 4$

Rearrange to get a quadratic equation and solve.

$x^2 - 4x + 3 = 0$

$(x - 1)(x - 3) = 0$

Therefore x = 1 or x = 3

Substitute your x values into the equation, $y - x = 1$ and solve to work out y values.

y = 2 or y = 4

Therefore the coordinates are (1, 2) and (3, 4)

Question 56: A

The gravitational potential energy of the ball at the top of the slope is *mgh*. The kinetic energy of the ball as it travels down the slope is $0.5mv^2$. The gravitational potential energy = kinetic energy, therefore:

$mgh = 0.5mv^2$

The mass values on either side cancel out to leave: $gh = 0.5v^2$

Thus we can substitute values into the equation:

$10 \times 5 = 0.5 \times v^2$

$\qquad 50 = 0.5 \times v^2$

$50/0.5 = v^2$

$\sqrt{100} = v = 10$

Question 57: A

As galaxies and celestial objects move away from Earth, the wavelength of the light they emit, gets longer as it travels towards us. Thus there is a noticeable shift towards the red end of the spectrum, when we measure those waves. Scientists are able to measure the real light coming from galaxies far away using telescopes that pick up and record this light. Using red shift we can tell which galaxies are further away and which ones are closer. There is another phenomena called blue shift, which is the opposite of red shift in that, we can tell which galaxies are moving closer to us as the wavelengths of those galaxies become shorter and therefore shift to the blue end of the spectrum.

Question 58: A

X-rays are able to pass through soft, less dense material, like skin, soft tissue and air to stain the x-ray film black. They can't pass through denser material like bone and thus the x-ray film stays white. X-rays are harmful with prolonged exposure as they ionise cells and cause DNA damage that can result in conditions like cancer. Radiologists or technicians working with x-rays wear lead aprons to protect them from excess radiation. Gamma rays are different to x-rays with shorter wavelengths that are able to pass through dense material and because of this, they are considered more dangerous than x-rays.

Question 59: A

$\frac{(16x+11)}{(4x+5)} = 4y^2 + 2$

$16x + 11 = (4y^2 + 2)(4x + 5)$

$16x + 11 = 4x(4y^2 + 2) + 5(4y^2 + 2)$

$16x - 4x(4y^2 + 2) = 5(4y^2 + 2) - 11$

$x(16 - 4(4y^2 + 2)) = 20y^2 - 1$

$X = \frac{20y^2 - 1}{[16 - 4(4y^2 + 2)]}$

Question 60: D

The first step is to multiply out $(3p + 5)^2$

$(3p + 5)(3p + 5) = 24p + 49$

$9p^2 + 30p + 25 = 24p + 49$

$9p^2 + 6p - 24 = 0$

Then put the quadratic into brackets.

$(3p + 6)(3p - 4) = 0$

Therefore p must equal -6 or +4.

END OF PAPER

FINAL ADVICE

Arrive well rested, well fed and well hydrated

The IMAT is an intensive test, so make sure you're ready for it. Unlike the UKCAT, you'll have to sit this at a fixed time (normally at 9AM). Thus, ensure you get a good night's sleep before the exam (there is little point cramming) and don't miss breakfast. If you're taking water into the exam then make sure you've been to the toilet before so you don't have to leave during the exam. Make sure you're well rested and fed in order to be at your best!

Move on

If you're struggling, move on. Every question has equal weighting and there is no negative marking. In the time it takes to answer on hard question, you could gain three times the marks by answering the easier ones. Be smart to score points- especially in section two where some questions are far easier than others.

Make Notes on your Essay

Some universities may ask you questions on your IMAT essay at the interview. Sometimes you may have the interview as late as March which means that you **MUST** make short notes on the essay title and your main arguments after the essay. This is especially important if you're applying to UCL and Cambridge where the essay is discussed more frequently.

Afterword

Remember that the route to a high score is your approach and practice. Don't fall into the trap that *"you can't prepare for the IMAT"*– this could not be further from the truth. With knowledge of the test, some useful time-saving techniques and plenty of practice you can dramatically boost your score.

Work hard, never give up and do yourself justice.

Good Luck!

Acknowledgements

I would like to thank all the UniAdmissions Tutors for all their hard work and advice in compiling this book.

Alex

About Us

Infinity Books is the publishing division of *Infinity Education Ltd*. We currently publish over 85 titles across a range of subject areas – covering specialised admissions tests, examination techniques, personal statement guides, plus everything else you need to improve your chances of getting on to competitive courses such as medicine and law, as well as into universities such as Oxford and Cambridge.

Outside of publishing we also operate a highly successful tuition division, called UniAdmissions. This company was founded in 2013 by Dr Rohan Agarwal and Dr David Salt, both Cambridge Medical graduates with several years of tutoring experience. Since then, every year, hundreds of applicants and schools work with us on our programmes. Through the programmes we offer, we deliver expert tuition, exclusive course places, online courses, best-selling textbooks and much more.

With a team of over 1,000 Oxbridge tutors and a proven track record, UniAdmissions have quickly become the UK's number one admissions company.

Visit and engage with us at:

Website (Infinity Books): www.infinitybooks.co.uk

Website (UniAdmissions): www.uniadmissions.co.uk

Facebook: www.facebook.com/uniadmissionsuk

Twitter: @infinitybooks7

Printed in Great Britain
by Amazon